Praise for *Open Wound: The Tragic Obsession of Dr. William Beaumont*

"The relationship between doctor and patient is hard enough to parse when both are in the same room. When one opts out, it becomes even harder. And of the gallons of ink spilled over the centuries in attempts at clarification, few efforts in recent memory lay out the frustrations and confusions and crystalline moments of grace better than Dr. Jason Karlawish's marvelous new book . . ."

—*New York Times*

"This is an excellent historical novel, so real that the biting winds of the western frontier seem to flutter across its pages and cool our sweaty brows. Within this, however, is something much more profound—a dark and gripping morality play about friendship, ambition, and the very essence of what it means to be a doctor. This should be required reading in medical schools. I will not soon forget this book."

—Jake Halpern, author of *Fame Junkies* and commentator for NPR's *All Things Considered*

"The ethical questions that envelop Doctor Beaumont and his patient are here laid bare for all to see—sliced through by Karlawish's sharp scalpel of finely-honed research . . . One can't judge this tale without pondering the possible experimental horrors our own bones and flesh might be enduring in our own time."

—Jackson Taylor, author of *The Blue Orchard*

"*Open Wound* is an enjoyable book that is not only a fascinating fictionalised biography of one of America's great medical pioneers, but is also an exploration of the complicated relationship between doctor and patient when it becomes transgressive."

—*The Lancet*

"This is a remarkable story, compellingly written, of how one man's ambition brings him both the fame he coveted and crushing failure. The propriety of a physician treating his patient as a living laboratory and as an avenue to personal glory is set down for the reader to judge. Beaumont was a man both desperate and delusional, yet one who advanced medical science albeit with questionable methods. A provocative read from cover to cover."

—Don Faber, author of *The Toledo War*

Praise for *Open Wound: The Tragic Obsession of Dr. William Beaumont*

"*Open Wound* is a fascinating novel about scientific ambition on the American frontier. Read this fine book for its meticulous reconstruction of nineteenth-century life, and for its evocative portrait of a medical researcher whose hunger for success leads him down an ethically dubious path."
— Karl Iagnemma, author of *The Expeditions*

"The story is fascinating on many levels, but it is Karlawish's portrayal of Beaumont's unstoppable, desperate, and almost dangerous ambition that takes center stage in this engaging historical account.... The story of the man with the hole in his side remains important, not only as a narrative of the early days of medical research and the emerging ethical issues, but as a cautionary tale and case study of that most American of personality traits — ambition."
— PRIM&R Ampersand

"In the grand tradition of the finest historical novels, Jason Karlawish accurately brings to life one of the most fascinating episodes in American medical lore, one that marked our nation's very first entry into the rapidly developing field of research on human subjects. We read here of inspired thinking, courage, ambition, betrayal and of one of the greatest conundrums — still with us today — in the ethics of medicine."
— Sherwin B. Nuland, MD, author of *Doctors: The Biography of Medicine* and *How We Die*

"Starting with the bare scaffolding of what is known, setting aside the flimsy particle board of legend and presumption, Jason Karlawish has crafted a carefully reasoned and beautifully written portrait of Beaumont and St. Martin. There is more truth — deeper truth — in this fine work of fiction than in many biographical writings on the pair."
— Mary Roach, author of *Stiff*

"A highly readable and plausible reconstruction of the medical and personal interaction between St. Martin and Beaumont."
— Richard Selzer, surgeon and author of *Mortal Lessons: Notes on the Art of Surgery* and the novel *Knife Song Korea*

{[OPEN WOUND]}

Open Wound

THE TRAGIC OBSESSION OF
DR. WILLIAM BEAUMONT

Jason Karlawish

THE UNIVERSITY OF MICHIGAN PRESS
Ann Arbor

First paperback edition 2013
Copyright © by the University of Michigan 2011

Published in the United States of America by
The University of Michigan Press
Manufactured in the United States of America
⊗ Printed on acid-free paper

2016   2015   2014   2013   5   4   3   2

A CIP catalog record for this book is available from the British Library.

Library of Congress Cataloging-in-Publication Data

Karlawish, Jason.
    Open wound : the tragic obsession of Dr. William Beaumont / Jason
Karlawish.
        p. cm.
    ISBN 978-0-472-11801-4 (cloth : acid-free paper) — ISBN 978-0-472-
02804-7 (e-book)
    1. Beaumont, William, 1785–1853—Fiction.   I. Title.
PS3611.A7836O64   2011
813'.6—dc22   2011020861

ISBN 978-0-472-03548-9 (pbk. : alk. paper)

for my parents,
Anne Wright and John Karlawish

In that land the great experiment was to be made, by civilized man, of the attempt to construct society upon a new basis; and it was there, for the first time, that theories hitherto unknown, or deemed impracticable, were to exhibit a spectacle for which the world had not been prepared by the history of the past.

———

ALEXIS DE TOCQUEVILLE,
Democracy in America

These subjects deserve better: a protocol that is not tainted with conflict of interest and is not tainted by our own professional agenda.

———

JAMES WILSON, MD, Philadelphia,
Pennsylvania, December 9, 2008

{CONTENTS}

{PROLOGUE}

August 1850
St. Louis, Missouri
Dear Alexis,
   *Without reference to my past efforts and disappointments, without
reference to expectation of ever obtaining your services again for the purpose
of experiments, upon the proposals and conditions heretofore made and
suggested, I now offer to you in faith and sincerity, new, and I hope
satisfactory, terms and conditions to ensure your prompt and faithful
compliance with my most fervent desire to have you again with me. With me
not only for my own individual gratification, and the benefits of medical
science, but also for your own and your family's present good and future
welfare.*
   *I propose the following—$500 to come to me without your family, for
one year—$300 of this for your salary, and $200 for the support and
contentment of your family to remain in Canada in the meantime—with the
privilege of bringing them on here another year. I submit this, my final offer,
out of the principles of Justice and Fairness.*
   *I can say no more, Alexis. This is my final letter—you know what I
have done for you over many years—what I have been trying, and am still
anxious and wishing to do with and for you. You know what efforts,
anxieties, anticipations and disappointments I have suffered from your
nonfulfillment of my expectations. Don't disappoint me more, nor forfeit the
bounties and blessings reserved for you.*
                                    Sincerely,
                                    William Beaumont, MD

PART I

The Taker Made Mad

{ONE}

June 6, 1822
Mackinac Island in Lake Huron, Michigan Territory

DR. WILLIAM BEAUMONT WAS AT HIS DESK in the army hospital when he heard the gunshot. It came from the bottom of the hill, in the direction of the American Fur Company's warehouses along the Mackinac Island harbor. He rose from his chair and stood before the small office window. The gate of the fort at the top of the hill was open, and several soldiers at arms ran down the hill. Within the minute, Elias Farnham, Beaumont's steward, flung open the door.

"Doc Beaumont, there's been a shooting in the company store. A young fur trapper's shot bad."

Elias held out Beaumont's surgical kit. Beaumont took it in hand, hefted the thing before he tucked it into his coat pocket, then together they ran down the dirt road to the American Fur Company store. The sweating crowd of fur trappers, Indians and soldiers stood in a golden halo of road dust as they tugged at their ringing ears. Dogs were barking. A child was crying.

"Doctor's here, let him in! Let him in!"

A soldier held open the door.

A ring of men, some standing, others squatting, surrounded a man lying on the floor and moaning. The smells of gunpowder and burnt flannel and flesh hung in the thick air. A young man, his clerk's apron blood-spattered, ran up to Beaumont. It was Theodore Mathews, the manager of the store.

"It's horrible, Doctor! Horrible! A shotgun discharged right here inside the store, and this fella took the blast close on."

Beaumont nodded. He knelt before the wounded man and reached out to lay his hand on the young man's shoulder.

"Easy there, lad. Easy. I'm Dr. Beaumont. I'll take care of you."

He took his surgical kit from his coat pocket.

"Elias, unroll my kit on the floor just to my left." He gestured to two men. "You there, ease out this lad's legs, one man on each leg. I need you to

THE TAKER MADE MAD

5

keep him from writhing about. Elias, you take his arms. And if you don't need to be here, please leave. I don't need an audience."

As he gave these orders, he was carefully stripping off the young man's red flannel shirt, using his jackknife to slice it away at the sleeves. The blast had torn a hole in the shirt. The edges of the hole were burnt, and the cloth was wet with the distinct smell of coffee and bits of what looked like breakfast meat and bread.

"Jesus," he murmured.

It was a horrible wound, the size of a man's palm, riddled with bits of fractured rib and cartridge wadding. Someone handed Beaumont a rag. He wiped away the blood and started to pick away the debris. The fur trapper moaned and coughed, and a protrusion of flesh heaved up, and the source of the coffee and food was revealed. The blast had torn a hole into the man's stomach. Beaumont sucked in his breath. Just above the injured stomach, a lobe of lung was caught on the ragged edge of a fractured rib. The man's breath bubbled through the blood that soaked the lobe. Beaumont used his penknife to snip the tip of that rib, then eased the lobe back into place.

"William, can I talk to you as you work?"

It was a voice as steady as Beaumont's.

"Yes of course, Captain."

Captain Pearce, the commander of Fort Hill and the Mackinac Island garrison, stood beside the doctor, watching him.

"I've got the assailant outside under guard. Teddy Mathews says he saw the fella set his gun down—set it down like it was a walking stick—and the lad here was right in the way of the blast. The balance of the witnesses' testimony is that this was an accident." He eyed the fur trapper. "A tragic accident," he said. "Look like that to you?"

"Hard to tell, but the shot's not direct. There's a bit of an angle to it, sort of upward and outward." He looked up and whispered to the captain. "If it was dead on, I wouldn't be needed here."

The captain's eyes narrowed as he peered at the wound.

"What on earth is that thing that looks like a turkey's egg?"

"Lobe of lung."

The captain grimaced. "Ah, Christ." He shook his head slowly.

It took the doctor twenty minutes to superficially clean the wound and apply a compress dressing. When he finished, he turned to Elias Farnham and ordered him to fetch a stretcher so they could carry the lad up to the hospital.

"William?"

Beaumont turned. It was Ramsay Crooks, the American Fur Company's principal agent on Mackinac Island. He was a large, red-headed man with a raw strength gained from some twenty years leading fur trapping expeditions as far west as the Oregon territory. Crooks gestured with his chin for Beaumont to step closer, and when Beaumont did he placed the length of his thick right arm upon Beaumont's shoulders and eased the doctor to a quiet corner of the store.

"You've done fine work with that Frenchie, William. Fine work. I always tell my sweet Emilie how lucky we are to have you on this island." He bit his lower lip, and looked in the direction of the young man. "You think that boy'll live?"

Beaumont considered the question. "He's not sinking."

Crooks grimaced. He tightened his grip.

"But do you think he'll survive the day?"

"In the war I managed wounds far worse than this. A few lived."

Crooks lowered his voice. "Let's just have him stay here."

"Here?"

"Here, yes. In the storeroom." Crooks released Beaumont and gestured to the door to the storeroom. "There's plenty of room, and there's always someone there. It's clean, dry and temperate. I've slept there myself some nights."

Beaumont frowned.

"Ramsay, I think perhaps . . ."

Crooks interrupted him. "Captain Pearce," he called.

The captain stepped over.

"I was just saying to William here that we can set the wounded trapper up on a cot in the storeroom. I'll be there at my desk to watch over him, and if I'm not, Teddy or one of the other clerks can see to his care, and William can check on him as he requires. Remember that fellow with the broken leg last year? And he was certain to live, and that's simply not the case with this one."

Pearce listened and nodded. Beaumont looked back and forth from the captain to Crooks. Speechless.

"What is it, William?" Captain Pearce snapped.

"Captain, the wound engages both lung and stomach, and I simply gave it a superficial cleaning. If he survives the morning, there's likely more to debride, and I'd rather manage that in the hospital."

Crooks smiled, and placed a hand on Beaumont's shoulder.

"It's a short walk down the hill, and you can come whenever you require. I'll even lend you a key to the storeroom." He spoke in a high tone, practically singing.

"But Ramsay."

Crooks tugged Beaumont closer to him. "William, you know as well as I do that I don't pay for these Frenchies to stay in the army's hospital. You start moving them in there, and then I've got some thousand men, women and children—white and Indian—living on that beach who can lay claim to a company-sponsored stay in the hospital. People with injuries far simpler than this man's. Think of the precedent, William. Think."

"I've plenty of empty beds."

"But you won't if you start fillin' them with the company's voyageurs and their families," Captain Pearce interjected.

Beaumont was incredulous. He looked around seeking an ally, but Elias was staring at his boots.

"Captain, this is an accident, not the war, and the lad's not dying. He's my patient now."

"Keep your voice down, Assistant Surgeon. I don't need a scene." The captain stared coldly at the doctor. "It's up to Ramsay, really. If he wants to pay room and board, I won't stop you from moving the lad to the hospital. A day costs little, and he ain't eatin'."

"I should say it's up to *you,* Captain." Crooks gestured to the wounded fur trapper. "That boy there is one of *my* indentured servants, and if he's anything like the lot of them, he owes me dollars against his indenture. But with a wound like that, even if by some miracle he survives the day, I'm never going to see that money. And now add to that a bill to house a dying man, not to mention the others who will come to expect the same. I can't run a charity hospital for the village of trappers along the beachfront. This doctor's *your* charge," he insisted. "He wears *your* uniform. And I might add that he seems quite busy stirring things up. Penning circulars about the expansion of the company warehouses and now standing here and telling me I've got to foot the bill for a lost cause."

He was speaking of a circular Dr. Beaumont had issued the other day to protest the company's plan to expand a warehouse onto the land where the garrison maintained a vegetable garden.

Beaumont stared at Crooks.

Captain Pearce exhaled heavily. The store was beginning to fill once more. They were being watched with increasing interest. Men were whispering.

"William, if Ramsay wants to pay for this Gumbo's room and board at the army's hospital, you can take care of him there. Otherwise, you care for him where he lays. That's what the army's agreement with the company stipulates. Be reasonable. I was in the war too. That lad's gonna die. You know that as well as I do."

Crooks nodded smartly. "I've heard enough," he murmured, and then stepped over to the wounded man. His eyes were closed and his breathing shallow. Crooks reached into his pocket and produced a handkerchief. He wiped his eyes and his brow, and then he slowly lowered himself to his knees and wiped the wounded man's brow. He looked at the men around him.

"Friends, this here is a terrible tragedy. It's sad to see one of the company's brave trappers wounded in the line of duty. He's like a fallen soldier."

Crooks shook his head mournfully.

"Teddy, you and the boys ease this young fellow onto a cot there in the storeroom. We'll set him right by my desk so I can watch over him and pray for him like he was my son."

TWO

THE VILLAGE OF MACKINAC ISLAND and the beachfront camps along the shore of Lake Michigan were astir with the labors of the day. The white walls of Fort Hill gleamed like a hilltop temple.

Beaumont was seated at his desk in his cluttered office at the hospital. His inkpot and leather notebook lay open as he had left them when Farnham came with the news of the shooting. His habit was to begin his day writing. The notebook served as both his personal diary and his professional record of cases. It contained notes on his travels and letters written and received. There were copied passages from the poet Burns, as well as his own observations upon the nature of man. Numbers and computations interspersed the written words, accounting his credits and debts, the former finally ahead of the latter. The notebook had become a collected record of his wealth, the chronicle of his ambition.

He dipped his pen and tried to resume writing. Ramsey Crooks was proposing to expand a company warehouse into the land the garrison used for a garden. The project threatened the plots of medicinal herbs and wheat Beaumont had planted. Beaumont drew a line beneath his notes about the garden controversy and wrote, *"Tended to a young voyageur at the Company's store. Shot into his left lower chest. Accident. Wound engages both lung & stomach, likely mortal."* He looked at these words, and then he set his pen down.

He gazed out the window at two men sawing a log. It was brutal, tiring work. The stack of raw timbers beside their saw pit would take at least a day.

During the war he could have filled pages of his notebook with cases like this young fur trapper, and for several weeks he had. And then he stopped. The war was fine training for an apprentice-trained surgeon with aspirations, but it was a cruel university.

After some battles, the wounded came without surcease, begging for relief. Some pled to have their arms, legs or even their heads cut off. Many of the chest and abdominal wounds, wounds like the fur trapper's wound, the doctors simply cleaned and packed as best they could to limit the egress of innards and left the men to die.

The doctors worked with increasing haste as the numbers of wounded multiplied. The maimed, gashed and dying lay upon whatever surface was available. The agonies of men dying or wishing they could die and the murderous grating of saws working through long bones filled the air. After several hours, their brutal work built several fly-covered piles of amputated arms and legs, some of the legs still dressed in stockings or boots.

He remembered one frigid evening in a ruined fort they occupied as a hospital, when the littlest of the stewards was clutching the amputated leg of a black man as he hesitated before the pile of white legs until Beaumont signaled with his chin to set it among the rest.

Even the name of the war was changing. The Second War of Independence was now simply the War of 1812. It was as though the three long and bloody years had become one, and the war was for nothing. It was just a single year when America and Great Britain decided to fight and then to make their peace. History was not a nation's diary of the facts but the selective forgetting of those facts.

Beaumont reread the lines he had written in his notebook, added the date and put away his pen.

"Goddamn," he muttered. In the war treating every man was impossible. But not here.

He looked at the nail of his throbbing right index finger. He had picked a rent into that nail until he tore it to its sore and bleeding cuticle. He snipped the errant nail between his teeth and spat it upon the floor.

In his walk back to the hospital, he had heard the murmurs, seen the men nodding, children wide-eyed and women whispering and pointing. The news of the plan to keep the young fur trapper on the cot in the supply room was spreading fast through the village, up the hill to the fort and throughout the camps along the lakefront. The more he reviewed that decision, the more he regretted his part. It was different when there were not one but one hundred men or more. When it was war and you were following orders. But then another thought struck him. What could Pearce and Crooks do if he were to carry the wounded man to the hospital?

For several minutes, he watched the under man in the saw pit struggle to manage the force the over man applied to the handsaw, and then he stood up with such force that he had to grab his chair to keep it from toppling.

"Elias," he called. "Elias!"

There was the quick shuffling of shoes across the gritty floor. The old man appeared at the door.

"Yes, Doctor?"

"Gather up my surgical kit. We're going to the company store to fetch that lad."

Elias did not move. "I thought the plan was that he was to be stayin' at the store? That you'd tend to him there."

Beaumont nodded. "I said, gather up my surgical kit."

WHEN BEAUMONT AND ELIAS reached the store, they heard the sound of men's laughter from within. Ramsay Crooks and three other officials of the American Fur Company were gathered about a table sipping from blue tin cups. Crooks was recounting his story of outwitting the Teton Sioux along the James River. A sunbeam illuminated a whiskey bottle at the center of the table. A haze of cigar smoke swirled above their heads. They turned when Beaumont entered the store.

Crooks blew out a stream of smoke.

"We didn't call, did we?" He looked at the others. The men shook their heads. Crooks motioned with his smoking hand to the open supply room door. "As you left him, William. Teddy's tending to him. Fancies himself some manner of hospital steward now."

The men laughed.

Beaumont went directly to the supply room. Theodore Mathews was wiping the man's face with a damp rag. He stepped away to give Beaumont room. The boy was awake, wide-eyed and breathing rapidly.

"I'm sorry, Doctor. I was just trying to help."

"No worries, Theodore. I'll take care of him now."

Beaumont lifted the boy's thin wrist and began to measure his pulse. It was racing like a snared rabbit's. The boy tried to speak, but the words were garbled. His desiccated tongue was shrunken to a dark nub at the back of his mouth, and his lips were chapped and cracked and bleeding. Beaumont hushed him gently with his forefinger to his own lips. He propped up the boy's head to give him water to drink, but the boy coughed and writhed in pain.

Crooks and the other men entered the room and watched Beaumont.

"Teddy here tried to give him some water but didn't know what was proper. Is this it then, William?" Crooks asked.

Beaumont gently set down the boy's head and then pressed the back of his hand upon the boy's forehead. Warm but not febrile. He inspected the tips of his fingers. Pink. He was not sinking.

"We need to move him to the hospital," he announced. "Now."

Crooks, his lips pursed, nodded to the other men, then said, "There were some voyageurs from the Blackfeather brigade here, what, just after you left. We could take him down to their camp along the beach. Be amongst his people. You could tend to him there, of course. More home-like, I'd say. I think it'd be best."

Beaumont did not take his eyes off the boy. "I said he goes to the hospital straightaway."

Crooks raised his thick red eyebrows. "You discussed this with Captain Pearce?"

Beaumont was inspecting the frame of the cot, testing its resilience. He looked at Elias. "I think we can use this as a stretcher."

Elias nodded.

"So then he's not dying as fast as the good doctor divined when he agreed to care for him here."

Beaumont did not turn to face Crooks. It was all he could do to contain his anger.

"No, not yet, Ramsay."

THEY USED THE COT AS A STRETCHER. Theodore Mathews at the front, Beaumont and Elias at the rear, though the boy was light and needed just two men to carry him.

The people they passed stopped their work. Some stepped out of their doorways or leaned out of windows, their arms crossed upon the sill. A woman gathered her three children close to her skirts. The dogs stared, their ears erect.

At the hospital they eased him into a bed in the corner, away from the north wall that in a winter storm was no better protection than a cotton coat. Beaumont gestured to the company's cot.

"You can take the cot back with you, Theodore. I'll have Elias return the blanket by the morrow."

Mathews shook his head quickly. "Keep the blanket. And the sheet. Keep it all."

"Thank you, Theodore. Don't you fret, you've done good work."

"Right then, Doctor. I best get back to the store."

The young clerk turned on his heel and ran out of the hospital. Beaumont rose and stepped across the squeaking floor to hang his coat upon a peg. He rolled up his shirtsleeves and turned to Farnham, who stood awaiting his orders.

"I haven't seen a wound such as this since the war. I'll need water, some of it boiled, some of it cool, and lint bandages, and at least one bottle of muriatic acid. He'll need more laudanum too. And duck fat for his lips. The water and the bandages first please, and after you gather the rest of the items start to prepare a carbonated fermenting poultice."

Beaumont drew up a stool and a low table, set his surgeon's kit upon the table, unlaced it and rolled it out before him.

"Quickly, Elias. Quickly if you please."

"Yes, Doctor."

The wounded fur trapper drew out his exhale into a long and low rhythmic moan except when he coughed. Then he would wince and cry, ball his hands up into fists and breathe rapidly.

Beaumont considered the task before him. The righteousness that had compelled him began to fade. In its place came doubt.

Without the operation, the lad would likely be dead by morning. The war had taught him that. He knew as well that this lad could very well die from the exertions of the surgery. To have carried the wounded fur trapper from the company store to his hospital against orders only to have him die would humiliate Beaumont. He could have managed the surgery in the storeroom. He'd operated in far more crude conditions. Crooks and Pearce would call him out as brash and intemperate. *Think of the precedent, William. Think.*

Elias Farnham returned with the supplies. "Is something wrong, sir?"

Beaumont looked up at his steward.

"No, I've all that I need."

He reached down and brushed the matted black hair from the young man's eyes and forehead. "I'm going to take away these dressings and clean up this wound. Mr. Farnham here will help me. Mr. Farnham is my steward. My name is Dr. Beaumont."

The boy was lost in his pain.

Though he was thinking of the agony he was soon to commit upon his patient, his manner of speech was a measured calm, a perfect equipoise between caring and indifference. It was a skill he had learned when he apprenticed under Dr. Chandler upon the residents in Champlain, Vermont. "*Aequanimitas,* William, *aequanimitas,* never let their sentiments and wild appetites get the better of you," Chandler would recite as a patient moaned and shrieked and wailed. "So too with your own," Chandler counseled his apprentice. "They obscure right reason."

He began to ease off the bloody dressing. It was a gruesome sight. Fractured bits of ribs, shreds of flannel with their edges burnt crisp and the pellets from the shot had worked their way loose. The sound of air bubbled through bloody mucus from the burnt margins of the lower lobe of lung. The skin around the wound was red and raw.

To keep the lower lobe of his lung intact when the young man coughed, Beaumont packed that space with lint. Using blade and forceps he began to pick away the flannel and shot and cut away the burnt muscle and skin until blood signaled he had reached vital tissue. Farnham had to forcibly pin the young man down to keep him from thrashing at Beaumont. His screams were piteous.

Beaumont said not a word. From time to time, he leaned away from the cot to allow Farnham to hold the young man as he panted in agony while Farnham murmured words of sympathy.

Within an hour, the enameled basin next to Beaumont was filled with debris, burnt tissue and blood-soaked lint. The fur trapper's pulse remained fast, but it was strong.

Beaumont wiped his eyes with his sleeve. He was exhausted.

"How are you doing, lad?"

His patient uttered a few unintelligible words.

"Say that again if you can?"

The trapper repeated the same words.

Beaumont looked to Farnham. "French?"

"I reckon so. I don't speak none of it but some bits, *bonjour* and *merci*."

The young man turned his dark eyes to Elias and spoke the same phrase again.

Elias nodded. "I believe I got it, Doctor. He's saying 'Alexis' or something like that, but I can't make out the rest."

Beaumont said, "Alexis," and the lad nodded and repeated that word and then another.

Elias slapped his thigh. "Alexis Samata," he cried. "He's saying his name, Dr. Beaumont. Alexis Samata. His name is Alexis Samata."

The fur trapper nodded slowly as he repeated the same words.

"Alexis Samata, I'm Dr. Beaumont, and this is my steward, Mr. Elias Farnham."

Alexis took them in.

"Beaumont," he pronounced the word quietly. "Beaumont," he repeated. He smiled weakly, and then he closed his tired eyes. He was short and skinny with impossibly long arms and thick hands. His chin and the sharp line of his jaw bore the smudges of a few days' beard. He couldn't be more than eighteen years old.

"I think he just might make it, Doctor."

Beaumont looked up at his steward.

The old man tried to smile. "You've done your very best."

"Thank you, Elias."

Beaumont rested upon his stool as he watched the boy's breathing even out into a steady, unlabored pace. His serial measures of Alexis's pulse showed a general relaxation of the high arterial action. He had survived the shooting, and now he had survived the debridement. The problem now was the summer heat. His experience from the war had taught him that within a day, two days at most, putrefaction and fever would set in.

{THREE}

WHEN WILLIAM BEAUMONT WAS A BOY, no more than five, an uncle rode in from somewhere out west on a roan horse outfitted with saddlebags that bore that man's initials hammered in gold. He carried a brace of flintlock pistols whose barrels were etched with mythical sea creatures, their smoky handles burls of high-polish walnut. On the pinky of his right hand, he wore a golden ring set with a green emerald the size of the nail of that same digit, and he was dressed in a soft coat that matched that stone. He sat before the fire steeped in drink, pipe smoke swirling around his head, and told his wide-eyed nephews of their ancestor William de Beaumont, who was named Earl of Warwick by William the Conqueror.

"There would have been land to go with such a title. Land and indentured servants. But centuries later we descendants, you and me, lads, are scattered hither and yon, toiling fallow earth, searching for our fortune."

He pointed at each of the boys with the amber stem of his pipe. He licked his dry lips.

By the morn, his father, rich in pride but poor in land and cash, called his brother a fop and a fool and ordered him never to cross his threshold. This brother's name was never again uttered, and in time it was forgotten. He told his son William that he was no namesake to any kith or kin, that there is nothing to a name but words.

"A name is just a name. Not some titular conveyance of talent or wealth and position. Our lives are as freemen in a free nation of democratic laws that rewards industry and virtue. Each man has to make his own name in this republic. Each man has to begin the world anew."

Some thirty years later, when Dr. William Beaumont arrived at the Mackinac Island garrison, his ambition of making his name in this new world seemed finally to be within his grasp. The previous surgeon had died, likely apoplexy brought on by opium and drink. The hospital he left smelled of mice, their little black turds wedged into the floor's loose seams. Bats inhabited the rafters. When Beaumont first entered the hospital, he could clearly see the afternoon sun shine through chinks in the walls. His steward, Elias Farnham, showed him the chalk marks on the planking floor he had etched to indicate where, exactly, to set pails to catch the rainwater.

In his first year on Mackinac Island, Beaumont lived alone in the garrison's physician's quarters, a four-room, pitch-roofed dwelling downhill from the hospital. Mrs. Farnham swept and dusted his rooms and tended to his meals and clothes. Like the hospital, his cottage was set apart from both the fort and the village. From his work table he had a view of the backs of the grand two-storied houses of Market Street, where the army's officers, Reverend James, Ramsay Crooks, and the company's managers resided.

One afternoon an injured hound dog limped to his doorstep. Beaumont mended his paw, named him Rex, and let the hound in to sleep beside the fire.

Among the officers and the officials of the American Fur Company corn whiskey was a staple. Swaying to their drink, they queried Beaumont, incredulous as they were at this new doctor's contentment to pass his vital years winter locked and celibate for near six months.

"Ya' frig yer own prick or what then?" a red-nosed Captain Pearce asked him late into a winter's evening of camaraderie.

Beaumont took no interest in his colleagues' advice on how to seduce an Indian girl. He was waiting for his betrothed, Deborah. She remained in Plattsburgh, New York, with her father, while the attorneys met discreetly to negotiate her divorce from Nathaniel Platt. Beaumont was devoted to Deborah and she to him. She had been alone in their childless home in the war-ruined city waiting for her husband, Nathaniel, to return from his travels. Nathaniel had no interest in the myrtle of Venus and kept at the bottle until dawn. There were stories of abominations he committed upon the stable boys. Then she had met Beaumont.

Beaumont took his drink modestly and passed his solitary evenings crouched over his worktable beside the fire. He read the histories of Mavor, Rollins and Antequil, Mackenzie's travels, recited Shakespeare and Burns, copied favorite passages into his notebook. He penned letters to fellow physicians and the leaders of Plattsburgh, filled his diary with passionate fantasies of Deborah. They soared upon the pinions of love. He wrote her long letters describing his life on the island and his plans for their family.

There was a calculated logic to his serving on the frontier. His solitary practice was like the company's monopoly on the fur trade. Suffer the island's isolation in return for a steady income and favorable prospects of advancement in the surgeon's corps.

AT TWENTY-ONE, he'd left his father's farm in Connecticut and traveled north to Champlain, New York. Cousins there had written of a brisk trade in goods to and from Canada. He worked as a shopkeeper, he speculated in hay and silk, and entered into politics, but his unyielding support of Jefferson's embargo act ruined both his business and his political careers. He taught school. In time, he grew determined to secure a steady income. He tried to learn Latin. He read a tattered copy of Thornton's *Philosophy of Medicine*.

Three years later, he collected what fees he could gather from the parents of his students, quit the school and crossed into Vermont and took up as apprentice to Dr. Benjamin Chandler. His debts were multiplying. In 1810, the War Hawks swept Congress, and by 1812 the United States was at war with Great Britain. President Jefferson's promise that taking all of Canada would be a mere matter of marching north became Beaumont's opportunity to pay off his debts, lay claim to land in Canada and make his name in the world. Three years later the fighting ended in a stalemate. Though he had gained neither land nor fortune, his surgeon's skills were now expert.

At war's end, he posted an announcement in the *Plattsburgh Republican* that Dr. William Beaumont, licensed to practice both physic and surgery by the Third Medical Society of Vermont, assistant surgeon in the Sixth Infantry Regiment of the Army of the North and veteran of the Battle of Plattsburgh, would commence seeing patients.

The ebb and flow of the suffocating fiscal anxiety of private practice reduced him to living in a slant-roofed room on the third floor at the back of Israel Green's United States Hotel. He had to duck a beam in order to step into the corner, where he had a small table and chair set before the shingle-sized window that overlooked the outer buildings. He swapped bottles of tonic for his meals at a regular table at the public house. For several months, he tried to walk to patients or negotiate a carriage ride, but the delay cost him fees, for patients soon found that either doctors Brown or Martin arrived quicker by horse, so he set down half the price in cash for a mare he kept in Green's barn and a promissory note good for the balance.

Nature itself seemed to conspire against him. The winter of 1817 kept snow on the fields and chunks of ice in Cumberland Bay until June. Then came a drought so severe that by autumn, acres of forests and fields burned. The air stank of smoke, and the evening sun hung red and pulsing, threatening like some great fireball overseeing the world's end. The few farmers who managed to plant crops lost much of them, revenues plunged, debts accumulated and commerce stalled. The merchants' wives ceased buying tonic, and the tally of fees owed to him multiplied. The preachers thundered that God was preparing the nation for the end times. He wished those without means would exercise discretion and limit their calls, but still they called, and often theirs were the most complex cases.

He kept a good pair of boots in high polish and a black dress coat and pants and stiff-collared shirt he wore exclusively for the Masonic meetings, the debating society and the meeting of the veterans of the Second War of Independence. He devised a rhyming game to learn the names of all the town's leaders and merchants. The monthly columns recording his debts and fees not collected grew together like two twisting serpents chasing his revenues collected. Some months, revenue led the chase; others, debt led revenue.

Finally, one summer Sunday morning in 1819, as the church bells rang, Beaumont sat shirtless and sweating at the tiny table in his cramped room, the flies humming, the pungent smell of horses carried in from the barn. He ceased tallying his ever-fluid accounts, set down his nib and decided he must return to the military service. The army had given a certain security to his life that the routines of private practice could not.

He composed a letter to Dr. Lovell, his commander during the war and now the surgeon general in Washington City. From merchants and leaders, friends and veterans of the war whose names and addresses he kept in careful alphabetical order, he solicited near sixty signatures on a petition to Secretary of War Calhoun and President Monroe. He gathered testimonial letters from the prominent and educated among these men that he was a man of first standing and respectability as both a gentleman and a physician. By autumn of 1819, on the eve of his thirty-fourth birthday, he set down one dollar and ten cents postage to submit his case to Washington City in support of his appointment as surgeon in the Surgeon's Corps of the United States Army. Then he waited.

Four months later, as Beaumont was patiently courting Deborah, Surgeon General Lovell wrote with the offer of a commission at Fort Hill on Mackinac Island in the Northern territories, not as a surgeon but as an assistant surgeon. Beaumont would have rejected it outright, for he was adamant that the commission he deserved was as a surgeon, but in his circumstances, he had no position against which to negotiate.

He explained his plans to Deborah one evening as they sat in the parlor of her father's inn.

"It's an opportunity for both of us. An opportunity to leave here and start again, together, as man and wife. The economic conditions are simply too harsh here, but I truly do believe in the future. At a garrison such as Mackinac I shall be the only physician, and that means we will have the income from not only my military work but also my work as physician to the residents and the American Fur Company. And the Indian office will surely want the Indians vaccinated against the pox. It will be remote, but it will be lucrative. And in time, as I accrue money and seniority and a reputation, we'll leave there, perhaps to return here. Return promoted to surgeon. Surgeon William Beaumont."

UPON HIS ARRIVAL IN MACKINAC, he set out to make himself a better man. At the end of each day, he whittled the tip of his carbon pencil fine and took up his virtue diary and recorded that day's tally of transgressions against the week's selected virtue and the preceding week's virtues as well. He had laid out the pages just as Dr. Benjamin Franklin prescribed in his *Autobiography*'s project for attaining moral perfection. A page for each of the thirteen virtues ruled with seven columns in red ink, one for each day of the week, and thirteen red-lined rows, one row a week. As Dr. Franklin instructed, Beaumont gave one week of strict attention to each of the virtues, beginning with *Temperance* and concluding with *Humility*. Thirteen weeks for thirteen virtues described precisely four cycles per year. Beaumont had timed his cycles to fit with the seasons, for he well knew how certain seasons tempted particular transgressions.

Franklin ordered these virtues with the logic that the prior acquisition of some might facilitate the subsequent acquisition of others. *Temperance* was first, as it procured a coolness and clarity of head so necessary when, as a physician, constant vigilance was to be kept up. This acquired, *Silence* would be easier. And so on through *Order,* then *Resolution,* followed by *Frugality* and *Industry,* making *Sincerity, Justice* and *Moderation* easier, and concluding with *Cleanliness, Tranquility, Chastity* and finally, though Beaumont thought somewhat oddly, *Humility.*

Beaumont deemed the *Autobiography* required reading for all American men, especially one such as him, a Connecticut farmer's son, who, like Franklin, was born into modest station and set out into the world with little or no fortune save his ambition. The *Autobiography* contained essential guidance for a man who intended to rise to even a moderate summit of his expectations.

But by the winter of his first long and solitary year on the island, as he charted his way through his third cycle of the thirteen virtues, he found Franklin's ordering of the virtues not as evident as they once had seemed. *Chastity* and *Cleanliness* were facile, but between them *Tranquility* continued to score blotches, and imitating Jesus or Socrates in *Humility* seemed difficult when faced with the likes of Ramsay Crooks and Captain Pearce. And how was Socrates different from Plato? And how to be both *Resolute* and *Silent?* The great Dr. Franklin offered little guidance on how best to balance the claims of one virtue against another.

IN THE SPRING OF HIS SECOND YEAR on Mackinac Island, after the thaw opened the harbor, he departed for Plattsburgh. Six weeks later, he returned with Deborah as his bride. She brought with her a few pieces of furniture and several crates of books and household goods. She ordered Rex out of the house and set up a semblance of a parlor in the one room that was neither bedroom nor kitchen. They had chairs and two tables, no couch, and just a single cabinet to display her books and the set and a half of blue-and-white china. Beside her husband's medical, history and travel books, his volumes of Shakespeare, she set out her favorite novels.

"There simply isn't space for the rest," she announced and directed him to store in the narrow attic space the balance of her books and her sheets of music, as there was no piano on the island.

Beaumont kept at his virtue diary. He was keen to eliminate the continued blotches against *Tranquility* and *Silence,* but in time, Dr. Franklin's exercises were neglected. This was not from transgressions upon *Industry.* His work caring for the soldiers and the employees and families of the American Fur Company and vaccinating the Indians steadily increased.

By winter, just after the New Year, Deborah showed signs of quickening. In June, just one week before the morning of the fur trapper's shooting at the company store, she labored four hours under Mrs. Farnham's care and gave birth to their first child, a girl they named Sarah.

FOUR

IT WASN'T UNTIL LATE IN THE AFTERNOON of the day of the shooting that Beaumont rested. He was famished. He desired nothing more than to return home to his wife and newborn daughter. The thought of them made him smile, but he felt an urgency to record his notes on the case of the young man they now called Alexis Samata.

He made a quick lunch of sausage and black bread as he sat at his desk sketching the shape of the wound, taking care to indicate the dimensions of the aperture into the stomach. He blew away the bread crumbs and stared at that sketch. This would be the kind of case he would never forget, the kind of case to share with his colleagues. There was a knock at the door; chewing fast, he looked up.

Elias Farnham stood at the doorway.

"I think you should come see something, Doctor."

"What's the matter?"

Elias grimaced. "I think it's best you see it with your own eyes, sir."

Beaumont followed Elias into the room where Alexis lay. "The lad was sleepin' like a babe until a few minutes past, and when he awoke, I took to feeding him wine mixed with vinegar and spring water. He takes it well enough, considering, but it's not staying in."

"Staying in? The wound's well dressed."

"Please, follow me, sir."

Beaumont sat upon a milking stool beside Elias. The enormity of the dilemma became evident. The little that Alexis drank did not remain in his stomach, but soaked out into the dressings and dribbled onto the bed.

"You see there, sir, how it all comes out that end."

Beaumont recalled the mess of food at the site of the shooting.

"What's wrong? Have I done something wrong?"

Beaumont touched the damp dressing. "No. You haven't done anything wrong. Perhaps I have." He began to explain the wound to Elias.

When he finished, Elias stammered, "You mean, his stomach's tapped open like a barrel with a bunghole?"

Beaumont nodded. "Yes. Give him some more please, Elias."

Beaumont gazed at the young man as he took another spoonful. A simple compress dressing was insufficient. To prevent this leakage, Beaumont knew he would have to plug the hole into the stomach with a carefully wrapped tight wad of lint, but while this treatment solved one problem, it would create another. When kept plugged, the hole could not heal closed. The stomach was one great fermenting vat. Even if Alexis survived the shooting, he would die of this hole and the leakage of its putrefaction onto the wounded tissues of his chest and lung.

"Try your best to give him what he can take. Smaller spoonfuls and pace them out a bit."

He sat and watched the older man patiently feed the younger one. It would be a horrible death. Unlike a limb where Nature afforded a joint to separate the morbid part from the whole, this kind of wound was to the very core of a man. He could not definitively amputate the gangrenous part. He could only cut away more and still more dead tissue and hope the wound would heal before there was no more tissue to cut away.

Perhaps, he thought, it would have been better to have left him at the storeroom, because when this man died, Pearce and Crooks would surely question whether the garrison needed a brash and disobedient assistant surgeon who made a show of trying to rescue a dying man. *The precedent, William. The precedent.* He thought of his sketch of the wound. Showing that to other surgeons would be perverse, an embarrassment even.

A WIND TOOK UP, swooshing through the high pines, rattling the windows, and within minutes, a yellow flash of lightning was chased quickly by thunder. "Oh my, now here it comes," muttered Elias. "I smelled it comin'." He stepped out of the infirmary room. When he returned, he carried a set of pails and began to place them on the floor over his precisely set chalk marks.

Within minutes, the hospital's roof rattled as if stones were being poured upon it, and drops began to fall into the buckets, at first singly like the slow beat of a drum but soon quickening to a regular flow. Farnham stood with his arms crossed upon his chest and admired the precision of his work.

"Say then, Doctor, what would it take to get us a proper new roof? That patchwork the soldiers did the other week did nothing." He motioned to a bucket, which was receiving a steady dribble of water. "You'd think with all the trading happening here they'd see to the funds for it."

"They?"

"The company, sir. Ramsay Crooks and his people."

"The hospital belongs to the army, Elias. It's Captain Pearce's decision whether we have a new roof."

Farnham turned and busied himself with his buckets.

"Their decision," he spat. "With all due respect, I think that lad's better here than layin' upon some rickety cot in that rat trap Ramsay fancies a storeroom."

"I do too." Beaumont used his fingers to comb back the hair that covered Alexis's eyes.

"Crooks's not just cheap but damn ornery. Just look at how he bullied you in that store, going on even about the garden. And Captain Pearce, why he's no more than some boot licker."

Beaumont rose from his stool. "I won't disagree with you, but I'm sorry I snapped at you when I called you to my office to say we were to go back and get the lad. The way I see it, in this world, men like you and me are the underdogs in the bottom of the saw pit, always halfway to what we deserve." He was looking over at Alexis. "Like this young fella."

"You did fine work today. You've got pluck. I've always admired that in ye, I have."

"I could use a bit of luck too. For him." He surveyed the room. The water stains upon the ceiling and walls had obtained new dimensions.

"I can keep that hole plugged, but with this dampness and the heat, I'd expect putrefaction will set into that wound by the morrow. We'll need to double our diligence with his dressing changes. Let me tend to some paperwork, but summon me promptly if he starts to turn for the worse."

The creak of hinges followed by the sound of wood slapping upon wood caused both men to turn as one. The door to the hospital opened, and a soldier in a rain-soaked oilskin slicker stepped into the room. He kicked the door shut with the heel of his boot, and then he looked at Beaumont. His face was rain slicked, and the brim of his hat was floppy and dripping. The man made a quick two-fingered salute.

"Doc Beaumont, sir, Captain Pearce sends me. Wants you up at his headquarters soon as you can muster ye'self."

BEAUMONT PAUSED AS he stepped out of the hospital. Drops of water gathered along the roofline, shimmered momentarily and then fell under their weight. He looked down at his boots and then at the rain-splattered mud. In just a few steps these boots would be mud coated to the ankles.

In the middle distance along the beach at the base of the hill, the rain-soaked sand had turned a darker shade of sepia. The storm had stirred up knee-high waves. He watched men hurrying to secure two errant canoes. Several naked children, their wet bodies shiny like seals, played along the shoreline. Since the spring thaw, in the field before the beach, the Indians and voyageurs had set up a crowded village of dirty tents and lean-tos, some displaying the fluttering symbols of their brigades on poles. A black feather. A roram hat. A *fleur de lis*. From somewhere there came the sound of a flute.

He turned and walked up the road toward the fort. His hospital stood at the midpoint of the hill between the village and the fort, like a kind of fulcrum between the powers of the United States government and the company. After he passed through the gates of the fort, he walked along a lane lined on each side by parallel lines of low blockhouses. The rain had turned the dust into pasty red mud that sucked at his boots. He stepped past deep puddles. Although the atmosphere was ripe with the odors of smoke, sweat, horses and garbage, it was the thought of Captain Pearce that caused his guts to tighten.

When Beaumont entered the captain's headquarters, an aide took his raincoat and shook it out briskly before he hung it on a peg, then admitted him into Captain Pearce's office.

Pearce was standing behind his desk with his arms outstretched so that he was leaning with all his weight upon the flat of his palms. His head was bent. He was reading something. The aide discreetly closed the door.

Beaumont stood three steps from the edge of the desk. His shoulders were rolled back, hands folded carefully at the small of his back, and his uniform coat buttoned to the collar. Pearce did not move. The chatter of the men in the outer office had ceased.

At the center of the desk was Beaumont's circular protesting the company's plan to expand its warehouse into the garden. It was kept unfurled by means of the captain's unsheathed saber. The saber was an elegant weapon with a lion-headed pommel atop a brass hilt, silver and ivory grips. The candlelight turned the deep bluing of its blade opalescent.

Pearce made a clucking noise with his tongue, and began smoothing his right hand over the circular in a gesture oddly reminiscent of a baker spreading flour upon a tabletop.

"What's up with that Gumbo of yours? He die?"

Beaumont shook his head vigorously.

"No sir, he lives. It's a complicated wound, but I was able to clean and stabilize it. As you saw, it engages both stomach and lung."

The captain raised his head.

"I bet you've seen worse."

Beaumont nodded slowly.

"I hear, Doctor, and I hope I hear wrong, that he ain't where we agreed to leave him."

Beaumont swallowed. "He's at the hospital, sir."

The captain's eyes narrowed.

"The hospital?" he yelled. A bit of spittle flew onto the desktop. "The hospital? What in the Sam Hill? Did we not agree he would remain at the store? Or among his kind on the beach? We all agreed upon a plan."

Beaumont shook his head. "I thought it best to have him near my care rather than in the supply room or in a tent on the beach," he said firmly.

"You thought it best to have him near your side," Pearce hissed.

Beaumont nodded. He stood like a soldier at attention.

"Did I not say, Assistant Surgeon Beaumont, did I not say as we all stood in Crooks's store that . . ."

Beaumont interrupted him. "I'm sorry, sir, but the duty of doctor is to his patient." He paused. "To speak plainly, I felt compelled to act. My professional duty demands it."

Pearce shook his head slowly.

"Well, I suppose that just fixes your flint. You don't leave me much choice now, do you, Doctor? What am I to do, send over a few soldiers to carry the man back to the storeroom or the beach? You've humiliated me. Do you understand that? Do you?"

He pointed at Beaumont, then he rubbed his eyes.

"You know Crooks won't pay a penny for that man's care. No reason to think he should once you moved the man to the hospital. *You.* Not Crooks but you. I just don't understand this. If you'd a come to me, we might have jiggled some cash out of that cheap Scotsman. But you didn't. So now if this Gumbo lives, I got that to worry about."

The captain began to pace back and forth behind his desk. He began to speak of loyalty and duty and the value of taking a man at his word. He spoke of reputation and shame. He invoked the nobility of the Romans and before them the Greeks. When he finished, he stood with his hands gripping the back of his chair. He held his head high as he regarded Beaumont, then sank heavily into his chair. He ran his forefinger along the length of the sword. Upon that blade was inscribed the motto *To defend constitutional liberty and property.* He gazed at these words, and then he looked at the doctor. His voice was now a low whisper.

"Listen to me. I don't object to you doctorin' who you see fit, when you see fit. It's who's paying for that doctorin' and room and board, that's my concern. Maybe Reverend James will have the town take him on as a charity case until we can send him on a bateau to Canada. Let me assure you that this will be in my monthly report. You may be the great doctor, but you're the insubordinate doctor as well."

Beaumont swallowed hard.

"It's my duty as commander. Didn't think of that, did you?" He was smiling. "Let me ask you something. You think he'll live?"

"I think so. For now."

The captain exhaled slowly through his nose.

"You think so. You all are no more precise than a blunderbuss at fifty yards. No more stunts like this. What's got into you, William?" Pearce gestured to the circular that lay open before him. "This circular." He read its title slowly. "*On the destruction of the garrison's garden and its consequences for the diet and health of the island's inhabitants.* You're quite serious about this?"

"Of course, Captain. It's my duty."

Pearce cocked his head. "Your duty? Your duty to stir things up over what you divine is right, never mind the rest of us."

Beaumont spoke, his tone confident.

"A proper diet is essential for the health of the garrison, and vegetables are critical. Absolutely *critical,* sir." He leaned forward. "It's clear from my correspondence with Surgeon General Lovell that there's a growing consensus on the matter among the surgeon's corps. The records we've assembled since the war, the experience of the war. I'm especially concerned with the loss of the land to grow wheat. You see, Captain, I think we can use that to brew a simple ale to substitute for the whiskey ration."

Pearce leaned back in his chair, and regarded his doctor as he stroked his mustache with one hand. "I respect your work, Doctor. I truly do. But sometimes I wonder if you and I are in the same damn army. Do you really think we can just do away with the whiskey ration?"

"We can't not try."

Pearce shook his head. He mouthed the words *can't not,* and then he spoke. "You know what I think of this?"

"No, sir."

"Never mind," Pearce said flatly. "I'm a soldier, not chief constable or gardener, and not a grogshop keeper. Four years ago I asked for a post out around the Dakotas. The Sioux are positively fierce there. That's some grand fighting. Positively grand. Can you temper your right to free speech? This kind of thing just stirs everyone up. Talk with me first. Can you manage that?"

"Yes, sir."

Pearce opened a drawer and produced a bottle. He glanced at Beaumont and swung his chin in the direction of the door. "Well, go on. Back to your Frenchman. Back to your wife and baby."

Beaumont was at the doorway when Pearce called out to him.

"Say, Doctor."

Beaumont turned.

"You got something for sleep? One of your tonics. I haven't slept right in, what, years. And don't just say stop drinking or dose me with some bitter purge." The captain gestured with the bottle so that its contents sloshed.

"I use the time. If I'm awake, I'm awake. So back to work until I tire."

"Until ye tire."

"That's right, sir."

"Well then, I'll give that a try then. Early to bed, early to rise. I bet that's your habit. Wealthy and healthy."

"Yes, Captain, Dr. Franklin recommended it. It has its many benefits. Good evening then, Captain."

"Say, Doctor."

Beaumont turned again to face the captain. The captain swallowed his drink, and stared at Beaumont.

"He's your patient, you say? Yes?"

Beaumont nodded. "Yes, of course, Captain."

"Well then, if they don't pay, the reverend and all, you got a charity case on your hands." The captain laughed. "Your purse," he added. "Not mine. Not the company's. *Yours*." Then he set the bottle once more to his lips.

FIVE

BEAUMONT RETURNED HOME AFTER DARK. His dog Rex trotted out from the shadows of the tall pines to greet him. Beaumont squatted and scratched the hound's soft ears. The dog sniffed his pants legs carefully, blowing and snorting, licked its pink chops and then moved off into the night.

"Evenin', Doctah."

Beaumont turned to face the voice. It was Edgar, one of the island's vagrant workers who carved out a living as a nightsoil man.

He walked past Beaumont with his long muscled arms draped over the length of a shiny pole balanced across his shoulders like some walking crucified. At the ends of that pole were suspended his stinking pails. He was stripped to his skinny waist, exposing an arcuate display of tattoos that covered him from neck to his navel. Those along his back were deranged by a lattice of scars.

Edgar had been on Mackinac since he was a boy, left over, some said, from when the British held it. Others said he was a deserter from the American army, a robber, an abandoned peg boy. At first, he worked as a low clerk to the company, but over time, as his tales grew stranger and more fantastic and more suspicious, the company assigned him increasingly solitary tasks until he settled into emptying the slop buckets. His dress became disheveled, his beard unkempt, and he seemed content to sleep under porches like some troll. He spoke of living on other islands inhabited by men with tattoos twice as elaborate as his. Sometimes he spoke to himself in a language of no discernable origin.

They tolerated him, made a joke out of him as he carried away their slops, until, one evening, he appeared at the officers' mess wet from the rain, near naked save for a kind of loincloth. He was reeling drunk. With his greasy locks flying about, he called them out as a lot of killers who were no better than the buckets of shit he slung. He fought them until he was bloody and broken and had to be tied down to a board. When they whipped him, he made not so much as a whimper, and then they left him for dead in the jail. Beaumont and Elias came that night, having tendered a bottle for the key to the cell. They carried him back to the hospital, calmed him with laudanum, wine and arrowroot, mended his wounds and cut his hair.

Company, garrison and village were united in wanting the man expelled. But Beaumont successfully pled to Ramsay Crooks, Captain Pearce and the Reverend James to drop the punishment. Mercy, he knew, would not move them. Instead, he argued that the man had value. Though his mind was diseased, his work was essential to the inhabitants' health. He convinced them Edgar was a strange but necessary employee to keep the air from turning foul and thus ward off the fevers.

"Evening, Edgar. Quite a rain today."

Edgar did not pause.

"Falls on us all, Doctah'. The just and the unjust."

"Yes, it does. It most certainly does."

"Fine work with that young trapper," Edgar said as he trudged on toward the woods.

BEAUMONT SLIPPED INTO THE SMALL BEDROOM in his stocking feet. He found Deborah asleep. The flame of a single candle upon the bedside table cast her shadow large upon the wall. She sat in a chair. Before her was the basinet where the infant Sarah slept.

He took up the candle and stood before the basinet with his palm cupped before the flame. He gazed at his daughter, now three weeks old. She slept with her forearms flexed and her hands close to her chin. Her tiny fingers slowly balled up into a fist. And then they relaxed.

Deborah roused. She looked at her husband. Her round face was framed by a bonnet.

"William."

He set down the candle and kissed her on her forehead.

"How are you?"

She closed her eyes. "Tired."

"How's Sarah?"

She leaned forward and looked into the basinet. It was a gift from Ramsay's wife, Emilie Crooks. The inside was lined with a goose-down-filled pillow covered in soft robin's-egg-blue silk.

"She's asleep. I fed her just an hour ago."

Beaumont reached into the basinet and used his pinky to brush a lock of hair from the child's forehead.

"Such a lot of hair for such a little girl. Look how even more has grown since yesterday."

Deborah rose from her chair, and they embraced.

"I love you, William."

"I love you too."

He shed his jacket and trousers, extinguished the candle and lay carefully beside her on the bed. She reached out and found his hand. Her fingers were thick, but their skin was soft.

"Forgive me, I'd have come home sooner, but Captain Pearce ordered my presence."

"Was he angry?"

"Angry?"

"About the boy. The one who was shot this morning at the company store."

"He's more a lad, I should say. Perhaps eighteen. How did you know?"

"Everyone knows, William. Abigail Matthews came calling this afternoon. She says Theodore holds you in the highest of esteem for what you did. You're the great hero of our small island. I'm so proud of you."

He exhaled slowly.

"Pearce has his temper, but all is in order now. The lad is resting, and I'm home now. Home with our daughter. I'd like to forget Captain Pearce with his rages and threats. Ramsay and his company."

The noise of a chat bird carried into the room as they lay side by side, gazing into the darkness.

"Ramsay Crooks can be so callous," she said. "You'd think the lad was an injured horse." She turned on her side to face her husband. "How is he? What's his name?"

"Alexis Samata. I think. His English is unintelligible. It's a bad wound, but he's alive and as well as can be expected." He yawned. "I did my best."

"I know you did. Emily said it was terrible, that you could see the man's very innards. Do you think he'll live?"

"That's hard to say. To be honest, I'm surprised he's still alive. The wound is deep and complex."

"Where is it?"

Beaumont took up her hand and placed it upon the spot on his body. "Into his side. I did the best I could. All I can do now is let nature chart his course."

"Of course you did." She stroked his stomach. "Did Captain Pearce punish you for moving Alexis?"

"No, no punishment. But you know how he can carry on. He yelled and hollered like a stuck hog that I should have asked his permission and threatened to report me as insubordinate, but then his bottle calmed him. In a way, I can't fault him. Mercy may be mightiest in the mightiest, but mighty men like Ramsay would indenture mercy herself to the highest bidder. Can you forgive me for being tardy?"

"Of course," she said. "You've nothing to apologize for. You did your duty."

He set his hand upon hers. "It's got me thinking of the war."

"Don't," she whispered.

"I know."

NEITHER ASLEEP NOR AWAKE, Beaumont listened to his wife's and daughter's sonorous breathing. How fickle is Fortune, he thought. The young man stepped into the blast. Had he not taken that step, he'd be asleep among his fellow voyageurs on the lakefront, and Beaumont would not be awake worrying about whether the man lived, the cost of his care, his own reputation.

He stared into the blackness. Upon him was the responsibility to see that his family rose up from their humble situation and achieved the life they desired. His father had left his family only debts. He desired to leave his family wealth. He expected years would pass before they attained their aspirations and sat before their own snug fireside in a carpeted parlor. The room would be lit brightly by a whale oil lamp and decorated with lithographs of American heroes. In time, they would have a piano and a music tutor for their children. He would hear the chime of the hour from his pocket watch, a watch finer even than Ramsay Crooks's. Guests would then rise from their seats to listen to Deborah on the piano. The men would run admiring hands along the top of a mahogany sideboard with its companion cellaret.

As he lay in his tiny cottage with his firstborn child asleep in a borrowed basinet, he worried whether he, the hero of this day, had pushed too hard for the French lad, whether he had sullied his reputation. He had done something noble, he thought, and yet the boy with the hole in his side might die a worse death than if he had done nothing. And if the boy died, he would be remembered as the doctor who disobeyed an order in a futile and vain gesture to rescue a dying fur trapper. Crooks and Pearce would have every reason to call him intemperate and insubordinate. But to set the life and the cost of the care of the wounded fur trapper upon one pan, and to set his aspirations for his family upon the other, and then to put on some blindfold and raise that scale and ask what were good to be done, that seemed wrong, even though it was the calculus of this day.

ALEXIS REACHED OUT INTO THE DARKNESS toward the pale light of the window. He gazed at the silhouette of his right hand, then set his palms together. After a moment, he crossed himself and lowered his arms. Slowly. It hurt to move. But he was not dead. His prayer had been answered.

When they came to carry him out of the dark storage room that smelled of tobacco and coffee and soap, the voice of the fat man who held all the company's indentures was thundering in his skull, and he reckoned that they would take him down to the beach and let him die among the tents. But they did not take him there.

They carried him, through the village, and into this quiet room that smelled of pine. He remembered the murmur of a man's voice like some priest, the taste of cool water. He dreamed of his mother, and then he awoke with the sound of rain and the doctor's servant at the side of the cot.

The doctor was not like the company doctors who ran their dirty, thick fingers over your gums like horse traders, thumped your back like a summer melon, checked your prick, pulled your ears, then slapped you sharp on your rump and sent you forward to the man, the cash box and the indenture papers.

He had been working since he was six. When he was twelve, his red-faced father had gestured to one of the two men he was told were uncles and said dully, "That boy is good to go."

He learned to plow. At fifteen he ran away to Montreal. He worked at a blacksmith's and then at a tavern. He lived in a basement and then in a barn. He mastered *vingt-et-un,* shot stones at the priests in the alleys beside the cathedral, stole from the warehouses. Then came rumors of British press gangs. He quit the city for the country, and in the summer he joined the migration south into the United States for the hay-making season. In fall, he returned north to chop wood, and in late winter, he tapped maple trees.

In the spring of 1822, he returned to his dilapidated home in Berthier. His father's stool was now empty. His brother Edouard served him a drink and told him he must meet the agents from the company. "That is some good money, and you need to get you some." Four weeks later, Alexis was pulling oars in a Blackfeather brigade bateau bound for Mackinac Island.

{SIX}

IN THE DAYS THAT FOLLOWED THE SHOOTING, Elias Farnham and Dr. Beaumont discovered that when they held Alexis curled up on his right side they could minimize the loss of the little nourishment Alexis would take, but in that position his pain was so great that he moaned and gibbered. He reached violently for their arms. Beaumont begged him to keep calm, to trust him, that this was all for his good, as he stroked his hand. But Alexis could not endure the pain long enough to eat.

Until the necrotic tissue was clear and the wound pink with vital tissue, Beaumont could not apply a compress dressing to keep the contents of Alexis's stomach from exiting. He could not properly feed him. He feared his patient would die.

Beaumont tended to Alexis at least three times daily. Elias was ordered to fetch him promptly in the event Alexis showed signs of decline. He personally managed the changing of each carbonated poultice to the wound and bathing it with a solution of camphorated spirits, water and vinegar.

Soon, a vigorous inflammatory response commenced. The wound just might rid itself of the necrotic tissue, thought Beaumont. But the evening of the third day began with the signs Beaumont had been dreading. Alexis began coughing, and within twelve hours he developed a thick cough and a hunger for air.

Beaumont practically lived at his patient's bedside. He wiped Alexis's brow with a cool wet rag and propped him up as he patted his back and held cloths into which Alexis hacked wads of green, blood-streaked phlegm. Once, he coughed up a button. For three days, Beaumont bled Alexis twelve ounces at a time until on the fourth day the arterial action began to abate. The fevers continued, and the wound became fetid with an odor so intense that it filled the room like a warm fog.

In time, the dead tissue began to slough away, and after four weeks, the fever subsided, and the wound's tissues began to appear pink and vital. The room smelled once again of dust and pine. Alexis was now so thin that you could count his every bone, but after Elias shaved him, he looked like a young man who might survive. He could tolerate the compress dressing, and his appetite was fair. When Beaumont and Elias eased Alexis to his feet, the young man rose feeble legged and wobbly as a new-foaled colt, but he stood and he took a short step. He extended his right hand, and he and Beaumont clasped hands.

"Thank you, God bless you, *mon* savior."

Beaumont smiled.

"You're welcome, Alexis."

Beaumont felt magnificent. Perhaps in months, even a year, the young man might fully heal. He imagined explaining the wound and its treatment to Surgeon General Lovell, imagined standing at the center of a surgical amphitheater as he presented this case to an assembly of surgeons. In the evenings, he found himself narrating that day's care to Deborah.

"You truly have earned the right to be called a great man," she said.

"I simply did my duty. Like countless other doctors."

"Precisely," she insisted. "Your selfless duty to your patient. Not to Ramsay Crooks, or Captain Pearce, or to any duty other than what your patient required. For that, you're a hero."

"Debbie." He was blushing.

In his solitary hours, when his thoughts wandered into his future, he imagined he was promoted to surgeon.

CALLERS BEGAN VISITING the young man who had survived the shotgun blast in the company store and the hero who had saved his life. Beaumont displayed his patient with great pride. He had Farnham dress Alexis in boots, britches and a new cotton shirt that Beaumont had traded the quartermaster for half pint of whiskey. They combed and cut his long black hair. They trimmed his curled nails.

A group of clerks from the company store who had witnessed the shooting, the manager who ran the warehouses and the laborers who worked at the docks came. So did voyageurs and their families from the camps on the beach. Debbie visited with the infant Sarah. Some of the visitors brought gifts. As the weeks passed, Alexis accumulated trinkets on his bedside table. One Sunday, Father Didier, the Jesuit, came up from his tent along the beach. He sat beside Alexis's cot and talked to him in French, then stood and prayed in Latin, crossed himself and touched Alexis's forehead. He left him a set of rosary beads made from dried betel nuts.

As the month drew to a close, Beaumont became preoccupied with worry. The costs of caring for Alexis, the bandages, the bottles of muriatic acid, the rations he was consuming, were all adding up. Before the summer was out, when Beaumont submitted his next supply request, the cost of Alexis's care would be obvious to Captain Pearce.

Some nights he did not sleep. He reviewed his finances. It was a cost he could not afford to bear, and yet to ask Captain Pearce to pay would not only humiliate him but also be futile. The captain would have fair cause to drive Alexis from the hospital and into a tent on the beach.

But this worry vanished when the Reverend James and a delegation from the town called to announce that the town would assume the cost of Alexis's room, board and care. "Charity," the Reverend explained, "is not simply a civic, but also a Christian duty." One of the men, who had been gazing at the water-stained ceiling, remarked to the reverend that they should take up a collection to pay for repairs to the hospital's shabby roof.

Beaumont grinned as he escorted the delegation from the hospital. When the men left, he turned to Elias and quipped, "The betel nut beads Alexis counts seem to have done their trick."

IN AUGUST ELIAS FARNHAM stepped in to the infirmary to tell Dr. Beaumont there were some visitors to see Alexis.

Beaumont did not pause his work rolling pills. "Show them in. I'm nearly done here."

Elias hesitated.

"Who is it?"

"Ramsay Crooks. Young Teddy Mathews is with him as well."

Beaumont frowned. He looked over at the other patients who lay upon cots near Alexis.

"Why don't you move Alexis to the cot in the side room and have them wait in my office. I'll see them there soon as I finish these pills."

Beaumont found Crooks and Mathews seated in his office. He took his customary seat behind his desk. Mathews was poker faced. Crooks was grinning. He reached his hand across the desk and shook Beaumont's hand.

"William, so good to see you. It's been ages."

"Ramsay, Theodore, this is like thunder in winter. It's not often I have the pleasure of the company calling on me here at the hospital. I trust all is well. How may I help you?"

"We've come to see the lad. I hear his recovery is nothing short of a miracle. And, I brought you a gift."

Crooks snapped his fingers and gestured to Theodore Mathews, who reached into a valise at his feet and produced a bottle.

"Bottle of my best Madeira," Crooks announced. He held the bottle before him; one hand gripped the neck, the other hand cradled the boot. "For you."

Beaumont took the bottle.

"Thank you, Ramsay."

"May we see the lad?"

"In a moment. Elias is moving him to a room where he can take visitors. He moves slowly. Alexis that is. Alexis Samata."

"He has a lot of callers?"

Beaumont nodded. "Voyageurs, some of your clerks. Last Sunday, Father Didier pronounced some sort of incantation over him and made a gift of some prayer beads, and the other day Reverend James called. Some days Alexis is the social center of the island."

"Reverend James?" Crooks's eyes narrowed.

Beaumont nodded. "He asked about the wound and how Alexis is recovering." Beaumont stood up and took three glasses from a shelf. "Why don't we enjoy this now," he said as he pulled the cork. "Some good news to celebrate. The reverend said the town will cover the cost of Alexis's care."

Crooks clapped his hands. "That is as should be. And when do you expect he'll recover?"

"Months, Ramsay. At least."

"It's that bad?"

"The wound's large, and there's still foreign matter lodged in the tissue. I'd expect he'll continue to extrude that for months. There may even be fevers again. And then there is the matter of the hole into his stomach."

"His stomach?"

"His stomach. He has a rent in the wall of his stomach that remains open. What's incredible is that the margin of those tissues has annealed to his chest wall with the result that the gastric contents spill out into open air."

Mathews was wide-eyed.

"You could stitch it closed," Crooks suggested.

"I could. I've thought of that. But that's not without its hazards. It may also heal by secondary intention."

"That's utterly fantastic, William. The lad lives despite a hole in his side. A hole right into his stomach. Imagine what you can see." Crooks elbowed Matthews. "What do you think, Teddy?"

Mathews mumbled a few words.

Beaumont set down his glass. "It is amazing, Ramsay. I've never seen a case like it in a man who lived."

Crooks took a long drink.

"It doesn't look like he'll be back to fur trapping this season."

Beaumont shook his head. "Not for a good while, Ramsay."

"That's too bad, William. Teddy here tells me I've got a three-year indenture on him, and Alexis owes the company forty dollars."

"How's that work?"

"It's not too complicated, William. He signed his papers like any free man and was paid out fifty at the start of the season. Up until the day of the shooting, he earned no more than ten dollars in work. So Alexis owes the company forty dollars of work. Or cash."

"Ramsay, why are you telling me this?"

"If ever he's well enough, I'll take him back."

"And if not?"

"Well, I'd hazard to say that the only men entitled to happiness are those who are useful. In short, he's a charity case."

Elias Farnham, who was standing off in the corner listening to this exchange, spoke up.

"Say then, Ramsay, is it in fact true that Mr. Jacob Astor, founder and president of your company, is a millionaire?"

Crooks faced Elias.

"A millionaire? When all the company's bills are collected, all monies owed paid out, all property fairly valued, perhaps yes, the sum of all his wealth is near to a million, if not more."

Elias whistled.

"You think that substantial, sir?" Crooks made a patulous grin.

Elias nodded vigorously. "Aye, I should say so."

"Well, I don't," he said plainly. "Frankly, gentlemen, I'm disappointed."

Crooks reached for the bottle and topped off his glass.

"Yes, disappointed." He set the bottle down. "I'm disappointed it has taken this long for one single, self-made man to wring a million dollars from the sweat of his brow. But I've every expectation that there shall be legions of Astors upon these lands."

"How so?" asked Beaumont.

"I expect the good doctor would want to know the secret."

Beaumont smiled. "I'm just a simple physician. Healing the sick may make for a steady income, but it's not the raw material upon which fortunes are mined."

"The way I see it, William, America is a great experiment. The wisdom of our founding fathers and the opportunity of our frontier liberate us from the shackles of old Europe, its bonds of aristocracy, of theocracy. In this free country, the true measure of rational man's potential may be fully realized. Money, William, makes money, and there is no more wealthy land than these United States wherein a man with pluck and a bit of luck can make his money. You know that before Jacob Astor ran the company, he owned a toy store, and before that, he was a baker. That's right, Elias. A baker. Cakes and loaves. And me? Had I remained in Scotland, I'd have been a shoemaker. It's what my papa did. It's what I would've done. And so on. Simple cobblers with no reasonable prospect for advancement. An aristocracy of simplicity. But *not* in America."

Crooks raised his glass. "To ambition," he announced. "Ambition! It is what makes money. And America is full of the raw materials for it and the kind of brave men who are willing to roll up their sleeves and make something of themselves. This is a country of beginnings, of projects, of vast designs and expectations."

"Points well said, Ramsay," Beaumont observed.

"Aye, but well done is better than well said. Mr. Franklin said that, I believe." Crooks winked at Beaumont. He looked over at Elias. "Say then, is the lad ready for callers? We brought him a gift. Show them, Teddy, what we brought for Alexis St. Martin. That's his name by the way, St. Martin. Not Samata. I know how their patois can befuddle. Go on Teddy, go on, show them."

Theodore Mathews reached into the valise and produced a package wrapped in brown paper and tied with twine. He set it upon the desktop with a thud.

"It's a Bible," he said flatly.

Crooks was excited. "In English. I doubt he's literate even in French, none of them are, but I thought it will give him something to do. People can read to him."

Everyone stared at the package as if waiting for it to move or make some sound.

Beaumont looked at Crooks. He began chuckling, and then he began laughing. "Of all the gifts! Of all the gifts! And from you!" He wiped his eyes with his sleeve. "I'm sorry, Ramsay, but this is *not* what I'd have expected. It is very thoughtful of you, though. Very."

Crooks was grinning. He elbowed Mathews. The young man tried to laugh.

"Don't mock me, William," Crooks said. "The spirit moved me! Think of this as a kind of celebration. Judging from the predictions you made in June, a reasonable man would say it's nothing short of a miracle this lad lived. Frankly, though my convictions tend agnostic—I'm Scottish, you know, and I've passed many years on the American frontier—I'm inclined to see divine agency in his case. Can you believe that, gentlemen, the very hand of God right here on our little island? A miracle some would say. Where's Father Didier when you need a bead counter? Well then, let's go see the lad with the hole in his side."

Crooks rose.

"Oh, and I nearly forgot. Memory's not as sharp as it used to be. We've cancelled the plans to expand the warehouse. Inventory's not as robust as we expected. So William, you can have your wheat beer and cabbages."

THEY FOUND ALEXIS seated at the edge of the cot. When the men entered the room, he slowly began to rise, but Crooks told him to sit.

"You're the wounded man. Sit. Sit, I beg you. And my, but you've lost weight. Look at you. Practically skin and bones. Why don't we send up a few pounds of salt pork for this lad? Can we do that, Doctor?"

Beaumont nodded. "If you wish. He's taking some solid food."

"Very well then. Teddy, see to it that we send up some salted pork for Alexis St. Martin. And some for the doctor and Elias as well."

Alexis began to speak, but Crooks silenced him. "Not a word of protest, lad. It's a gift. You are a most fortunate man, you know that? Most fortunate." He spoke in French for a few moments.

Alexis nodded. "*Il est mon saveur.*" He pointed at Beaumont.

"Yes indeed he is," Crooks said. "Your savior. We miss you at the store, Alexis. Your singing." Crooks turned to Beaumont and Farnham. "You know, gentlemen, he's got a talent for song? That's right. And his English isn't half bad." He turned back to face Alexis.

"Soon as you're well enough, we'll have you back and singing. But until then, you rest and get your strength back. I've a gift for you. *Un cadeau.*" Crooks held out the package with two hands. Alexis reached out to take it but then winced and withdrew his hand.

"His chest's still quite sore." Beaumont said.

Elias took the gift.

"Here now, Alexis. I'll put this back by your bedside, we can open it later."

The four men stood gazing at Alexis. A tinkling of musical chimes broke the silence. Crooks reached into his vest pocket for his gold-cased pocket watch.

"*Tempus fugit,* Teddy. We must get back to the store." He returned the watch to his vest and smiled at Alexis. "Well then, Alexis, time is money, and we've got chores to tend to. Good day to you."

"Good day, Mr. Crooks. Thank you for the gift."

After Crooks and Mathews left, Elias and Beaumont returned to help Alexis to his cot. Beaumont began to whistle.

"Happy, sir?" Elias asked.

Beaumont chuckled.

"The gods are answering all our prayers."

SEVEN

ALEXIS'S ROBUST ENDURANCE in the face of pain astounded Beaumont. He could not sit up without obvious distress from the motion of the fractured ribs, and each cough sent lacerating pains through his chest. Still, his smile was warm, and his appetite was improving.

To better treat these pains, Beaumont designed, commissioned and oversaw the armorer's production of a tiny saw. Its thin brass blade had teeth as fine as sand and sharp as a lizard's teeth. Its haft was a polished mahogany that the armorer included at no extra expense, for he much admired Beaumont's ingenuity. With just three strokes of this blade, Beaumont deftly sawed away a rotting, fractured rib.

Elias Farnham cut Alexis a length of a cane from an ash sapling, and Alexis used this to steady himself as he walked across the hospital floor, the cane in one arm, the other wrapped around Elias's waist. The two of them moved like frail partners at a barn dance. In time, he stepped outdoors to sit on the bench overlooking the garden. He talked with the soldiers and voyageurs who stopped to see the miracle man. He raised his shirt to show them the wrapping of bandages. He was not shy. His collection of belongings beside and beneath his cot soon included objects he'd gathered outdoors. He took to whittling decorations along the length of his cane.

"He's got a talent there, Doctor," Elias remarked as he displayed the complex design of rosettes, curlicues and fantastic birds.

BY EARLY OCTOBER, three months after the shooting, summer was fast vanishing. Days were shorter but the light brighter, as if the sun were burning more intensely in a futile gesture to stall the onset of winter. The agents from the American Fur Company, and the American soldiers and their officers, prepared Mackinac Island for the interminable months of frozen isolation. The brigades of voyageurs and Indians dismantled their tent and lean-to village along the lakeshore and embarked in their bateaux and canoes and paddled north to Canada or south to the Michigan Territory to take shelter in the pine and hardwood forests. The white children returned to school.

Alexis's days had settled into a routine which began when Beaumont stepped into the infirmary of the ramshackle hospital carrying his basket of medical supplies.

"Good morning, Alexis."

He smiled as he watched Alexis yawn and rub the mount of his palms against his eyes.

"Good evening, *mon* Dr. Beaumont." Alexis laughed. "Good morning. Morning." His accented English ran hard on the *d*'s, swallowed the *r*'s.

Still sore from his wound, Alexis lay flat upon his back, gathered his nightshirt under his armpits, then folded over the thin blanket to reveal his abdomen swaddled with the bandages Beaumont had applied the previous evening. Beaumont took care to wrap the bandages tightly around Alexis's torso from his chest to his navel. To keep them in place, he passed a final wrapping like a Sam Browne belt, across his right shoulder. The bandages themselves revealed the progress of the wound's healing. It had been at least four weeks since the outer layer showed the ruddy stain of discharge.

As usual, Alexis gazed straight up at the ceiling, waiting patiently, blinking. "Madame Beaumont, she is well?"

"She's well. Quite well."

Alexis nodded and smiled. "Little Sarah?"

"Very well, thank you. They wish you well too. Now please, Alexis, if you could just lie still as usual."

Beside Alexis's cot Beaumont placed the simple brown wicker basket that held bandage rolls, his surgeon's pocket kit and a bottle of diluted muriatic acid he had gathered from the supply room. He sat on the edge of the bed, just inches from Alexis. The bed frame creaked as it always did.

Beaumont took his surgeon's kit from the basket, unrolled it on the mattress, took up his jackknife and set to work methodically cutting away the dressings. Someone whistled as he passed close to Alexis's window, and Beaumont hummed a few bars of that tune. He found himself tapping his foot to the timing of the blacksmith's hammer.

He folded away the sliced bandages to reveal a wad of carefully packed bandages the size of a tea saucer. The skin around the wound was still inflamed but no longer grossly purple. It blanched under the gentle press of Beaumont's thumb. He had not bled Alexis in over eight weeks.

He began to peel away the lint packing, and with that packing now removed, the pink ruggated puckering of the inner lining of stomach bloomed through the wound like some large rose. Alexis coughed, and the bloom expanded, glistening and covered with a limpid fluid, uniformly spreading over its whole surface and trickling to the edges of the wound. Beaumont gazed upon this display for some moments, then applied three fingers of gentle pressure to the center of the bloom, and it slowly depressed into the blackness of the space that was Alexis's stomach. An amazing sight each time he witnessed it.

Beaumont folded a clean lint bandage into a square, soaked this with muriatic acid and began to wipe the edges of the wound and the track where Alexis once had a fifth rib. In time, Beaumont thought, all in time, this wound will close, and I will have a case worthy of the *Medical Recorder.*

Alexis coughed again. A bit of meat, chewed, but unmistakably meat, popped out from the aperture and onto the bandages, and a slow trickle of gastric juice flowed out from the lower margin of the wound.

Beaumont picked up the meat and inspected it. He had instructed Alexis to keep an empty stomach to prevent just such soiling of the wound during morning dressing changes. Now he held in his hand the evidence that Alexis had stolen a meal some time in the early morning hours. He was disobedient to be sure, yet this clandestine meal also was another sign of his slow, but now certain recovery.

Alexis laughed and muttered in French. Beaumont had seen food in just this state before. There was nothing unique about this morning and this piece of meat.

As he held the partly digested piece between his thumb and forefinger and gazed at the wound, two facts came together for him. He felt as he had that morning some ten years past when he first stepped into his assigned hospital tent at the camp in Plattsburgh. Or when taking calls as apprentice to Dr. Chandler. It was the same sense in his guts and rush of blood to his head as when he was a boy jumping from the barn's rafters into the hay pile.

For weeks he had observed that the hole into Alexis's stomach gave off no odor or other evidence of putrefaction. Perhaps the cavity did not work as he had been taught, like a barrel to churn and ferment food, but in some other and, it seemed, more elegant manner. The action of the muriatic acid with which he painted the wound to cleanse it and stimulate healing was the same as the action of the stomach upon this piece of salt pork. The action was like a solvent upon the flesh, a solvent that affected a steady dissolution of the tissues. The stomach was perhaps not as he and so many of his colleagues had thought it to be, some grinding bag or fermenting vat. It was some manner of chemistry, like an alchemist's trick that made flesh disappear.

On this morning, an idea kindled not reason's ordered plans, but desire laid to make the taker mad.

Alexis was his patient, of course, but he could be something else too. Beaumont could not conjure the proper word, but whatever the word, on this morning he realized that this man, this wound, was his window to discovery.

Wondrous discoveries. Discoveries of the secrets of digestion and diet that would rival the work of the famous Parisian physicians. There wasn't another proper doctor within hundreds of miles, a situation conducive not

THE TAKER MADE MAD

43

only to a steady and good income but now also the discovery of this treasure. It was his, and it was simply waiting to be explored and written into a book. It was like the vast Western lands that President Jefferson purchased and captains Lewis and Clark charted and from which the American Fur Company extracted profits. The unknown was waiting to be known, and once known, rewards would follow. Promotion to surgeon secured, election to medical societies. He would erase the humility of his medical training as an apprentice and the condescension of the medical college graduates. His reputation would be solid and preserved for posthumous time.

He shook his head like a drinker who'd swallowed more than his fill.

I am a doctor, not a scientist, he thought. This was work he had no sense of how to do, where to begin or how to finish, before the wound fully healed and sealed its secrets. How would he convince Deborah of the worth of this sacrifice of time and money? And if it was ever done, whatever it really was, he had no idea how to sell it. The idea was swallowed bait, a folly even.

"Goddamn," he muttered.

Alexis grew concerned.

"What is it? Is there problem? A type of what you call, what you call, pains. *Oui?*" His smile had vanished.

Beaumont tried to calm his patient. He began to quickly wrap the bandages into a wad.

"Nothing's wrong, Alexis. Nothing at all. You're doing well. Truly, yes, all is well." He reached out and embraced Alexis. He smiled as best he could. "You're the very model of recovery."

Alexis wrinkled his eyebrows, then relaxed and returned his doctor's smile like a moon reflecting the light of its sun but ignorant of the nature of fire that kindled that illuminating light. He spoke in unusually clear English.

"No, my Dr. Beaumont, I am your miracle."

THAT EVENING AS BEAUMONT was writing in his notebook, Deborah, dressed in her nightshirt, slippers and cap, stepped behind him. She placed her hands tenderly upon his shoulders. Beaumont startled.

"Penny for your thoughts," she said.

He set down his quill. "Just reviewing accounts."

"You seem quiet tonight."

He turned to face her.

"A bit of dyspepsia, but I'm well. Don't wait up for me."

⁌[EIGHT]⁍

HE RETREATED TO HIS OFFICE AND HIS BOOKS and notebook. He read with his elbows on his desk, his head between his hands. Some days he read till dark.

On one of these evenings, a voice roused Beaumont. Brevet Major Hardage Thompson stood at the doorway. He held his hat in his hands. Beaumont smiled and gestured to a chair.

"Hardage, I didn't hear you enter. What is the hour?"

"It's round six. I saw your light on and wondered what has you burning midnight's oil. I see you're thoroughly absorbed over your text."

The major was a squat-framed man, one of the oldest officers at Fort Hill, with just a few tufts of close-shorn gray hair that formed a tonsure about his round head. Among all of the officers, he was Beaumont's closest friend. A veteran of the war, like Beaumont, he shared the bond of humble origins and a reputation built solely on his own hard work. The major had risen to his rank from his enlistment some twenty-five years ago as a common private.

Thompson took his seat. Beaumont looked down upon the much-worn volume open before him. His notebook was propped open beside this by means of a stone he had gathered in his explorations of the island. The tip of his right forefinger was stained with ink. He turned a page idly.

"I was reading Brown's *Elementa Medicinae* on the process of digestion," he explained. "It's truly limited. Do you know some maintain that the stomach is not a grinder and fermenter—as I've always thought—but instead that it works by a kind of chemical process?"

Thompson nodded politely. He looked about the office. "It seems only yesterday that the Frenchman was all but certain for dead. And now he walks. What you've done is nothing short of a miracle."

Beaumont chuckled. "You sound like the Reverend James. Our good cleric seems to suggest that my skill had little influence in Alexis's recovery. Never mind my years of apprenticeship. Never mind the years at war. As if I'm some Catholic conjurer."

"How is the lad?"

"Well, though still recovering. The wound's complicated, very complicated, and he has that hole that's slow to heal."

THE TAKER MADE MAD

45

"Into his stomach."

Beaumont nodded. "Directly."

Thompson looked at the copy of *Elementa Medicinae*. Beaumont followed his gaze. "It's made me curious, I confess."

Thompson gestured to the text. "I'm sure you'll find something in there to help you close that hole up. I tell Sally often how we're so fortunate to have a surgeon of your skills and intellect at this garrison."

"Assistant surgeon, Hardage. Assistant." Beaumont held up the index finger of his right hand to punctuate the point. "But thank you. Truly, it's my duty, though I'm proud of what I've done. You heard about the little saw I commissioned?" He smiled.

"Aye."

"Not bad for an apprentice-trained assistant surgeon."

"The one before you saw his duty largely at the grog shop."

Beaumont rubbed his eyes. He looked out the window at the shadows of the dilapidated outer buildings. "And he was a post surgeon and university trained as well. Between Captain Pearce and Ramsay Crooks a man has got to keep his wits," he said.

"Who pays for the Frenchman's care?"

Beaumont's eyes narrowed. "You've heard something?"

"Pearce grumbles."

"Not a surprise." Beaumont hesitated. "You know, on the day of the shooting Crooks wanted Alexis to remain in the store, and Pearce supported him. Of course. They said that to have Alexis in the hospital would set a precedent for other fur trappers. I reluctantly agreed, but then my conscience caught up to me. Elias and I went back and took him. Pearce gave me a tongue-lashing for that." He faced Hardage. "I'm pleased I took Alexis to the hospital. It's a decision I don't regret for a minute. If there is some good to come out of that war, it's what we learned in the care of such wounds as Alexis's. But never the mind. Whatever stain my reputation may have suffered, I'm confident subsequent events have washed it away. Pearce will forget, and Ramsay made his peace with me."

Beaumont brightened. "Look there!" He gestured to the bottle of Madeira. "He even gave me a gift. And Reverend James himself stood in this office and told me the town has taken Alexis on as a charity case."

"What if they refused?"

"Refused?"

"What if the town refused to support the lad? There're rumors that the money's running out. I'm sure they're afraid of having to take on others as well."

Beaumont drummed his fingers on the desktop. "Well then, I'd hazard Alexis would be in trouble. I'd do what I could. I can take on the occasional charity case for a spell. You know, rob Peter to pay Paul for hospital supplies. Mind you, I learned my lesson with that kind of thing back when I was in private practice in New York. I nearly lost my shirt then. With Alexis, I'd hazard it's the cost of the room and board that's the rub."

He became lost in thought.

"What's wrong, William?"

Beaumont's mind was racing with the figures of the costs of Alexis's care. "Nothing, I was just thinking how I doubt Debbie would allow it."

"Allow what?"

"Allow me to take Alexis on as my own charity case. Why, it's only this year that by my own pluck, and a bit of luck too I confess, I've finally freed myself from the shackles of my many debts. And now we have the baby." Beaumont smiled. "She's such a delight. I tell you, the other day she smiled at me and laughed. She's going to be a fine and charming woman, as striking as her mother in every respect." He eased back into his chair. "I must think of my family. Our funds are limited."

The two men sat in quiet company. The sound of children playing at a game carried in. Beaumont turned a few pages of the book. Thompson tossed his cap around the outstretched fingers of his left hand, ran his fingers through his thin gray hair. He surveyed the collections of books, the stacks of the *Eclectic Repertory,* an arrangement of pottery medicine containers ordered by size and with paper labels of their contents. Upon the desk there were Beaumont's notebooks, a basket with stones and another with curios of wood and shells, and two thumb-sized beetles mounted upon a board the size of a playing card. Thompson's attention settled upon a sealed jar that held a collection of bile stones. He took it up to more closely inspect its emerald contents. When he spoke, he was incredulous.

"You'll never fathom what Lieutenant Russell has told me."

Beaumont closed his text. "What now?"

"He says he and Lieutenant Morris decline to testify against your malingerer Lieutenant Griswold."

"Decline?"

"Recant. Withdraw. Something in that manner." Thompson picked up the pace of his cap's circular motion. "They want to withdraw any complaint against Lieutenant Griswold. I suppose they wish I'd drop all charges of his shirking his duty."

Beaumont leaned over the desk. "But why?"

Thompson shrugged. "Collusion among the ranks? They're all academy men, you know, a kind of club I'm not a member of. I truly can't say. I pressed each for a reason, and they maintain that Lieutenant Griswold was ill, now he's better and no harm was done. They regret their complaint."

Beaumont grimaced. "No harm in malingering to shirk duty?" he insisted. "Truly not."

"Truly so. Of course Griswold's court-martial proceeds with or without their testimony. We have your medical report to substantiate the charges."

FOR MUCH OF THE MONTH OF JUNE, the case of Lieutenant Edmund B. Griswold had occupied Beaumont. For three weeks, the young lieutenant had recited a litany of complaints that began with a series of pains in his feet, the left one greater than the right, but soon were general. One he called his cold bone pain. This, the man complained, lay deep in his bones. He shivered when he spoke of it. The other was more in his skin and flesh. Stomach cramps came and went. And there was also a rash.

The lieutenant insisted he remain upon the sick roll, and he passed his days on his cot reading novels. It was after Major Thompson's third petition to Dr. Beaumont to see the man that Beaumont made his final diagnosis.

His *methoda medica* was elegant. He proved that the young lieutenant had lied about taking his prescribed medicine. Beaumont had told Griswold that the neatly folded brown paper packet was a gentle stimulant. In fact, it was calomel, a medicine designed to produce certain vomiting.

When Beaumont returned to check on his patient, he found the young lieutenant on a bench enjoying the last of the day's sun. His copy of *Sentimental Journey* lay open beside him. He claimed some, though not entire, improvement after taking the medicine, and yet his jaws, mouth and general appearance, his history and the collaborating history from lieutenants Russell and Morris, concurred upon one single and certain conclusion. Though Lieutenant Griswold claimed he had taken the medicine prescribed by doctor's orders, he clearly had not.

The man was a malingerer.

Beaumont explained the diagnosis to the major and his lieutenants, Russell and Morris.

"A sick man who calls for medical attention and submits to examination takes his prescribed treatment. A well man who's using physical complaints to shirk military duty, that man does not take the dose. And in this case, that man is Lieutenant Edmund B. Griswold."

That very day, Beaumont struck the lieutenant's name from the sick roll, and Major Thompson brought up court-martial charges, and the man was sent to the jail for failure to follow orders, disobedience and insubordination.

MAJOR THOMPSON'S NEWS that the lieutenants Russell and Morris now refused to testify against their fellow lieutenant irked Beaumont. "Can't you compel them to testify?" he asked. "You're their commanding officer."

"I am their commander, William, yes I am, but I can't compel them. But that's of little concern. We have the solid facts of your report. Lieutenants Russell and Morris wish to use sentiment and feeling to counter medical science, best of fortune to them."

Beaumont was frowning as he reached for his notebook and flipped back several pages.

"I saw him outside his quarters, in his shirtsleeves with no other protection than his usual apparel. If Lieutenant Griswold had taken that medicine as I directed him, he would have had swelled jaws and a sore mouth. He'd not have been seated before the plate of boiled beef and potatoes lieutenants Morris and Russell saw him eating earlier that day. Finally, when I inspected him, I saw not one sign consistent with the dose of calomel I prescribed, and neither did he complain of soreness in his mouth or his jaws. That, Major, is, I submit, the scientific proof."

"I don't doubt you, William."

Beaumont thumped the tips of his thumb and forefinger on the desk. "The plain and unvarnished truth. If he took his dose as I instructed him, and as he claimed he did, it would have exerted violent effect upon him. He would have begun puking within minutes. It's an experiment designed with the simple elegance to prove him out as a malingerer. The proof is evident."

Beaumont gestured to his books and journals.

"I have issues of the *Eclectic Repertory* that speak objectively and scientifically upon the diagnosis of malingering. It's seen not infrequently. A sick man takes his prescribed treatment, but a well man does not. I've an authoritative record of a case from a garrison in the Florida territory that used scarification by cupping to great effect. I think my methods more humane as they will leave no scar upon his person, though his reputation, I can hazard, will suffer certain blemish."

Beaumont's face had turned a deep red. "And what is a man but his reputation? Glass, china and reputation, Hardage. They are easily cracked and never well mended. Franklin said that." He pointed to his friend and nodded. "Take reputation away, and all that remains is the bestial part."

The major was listening intently to Beaumont.

"You'll wring no argument out of me on the matter, William. The facts you submit are clear. Clear scientific facts. And Dr. Franklin's wisdom is true. 'Tis disappointing the lieutenants decline to testify, or even if ordered, will insist they were wrong. But no worries, William. The facts will win out. They always do."

Beaumont frowned. "I hear his father's a senator," he said.

Thompson shook his head. "Was. Now the man's a judge. In Connecticut, I think. He comes from an old Connecticut family."

"Well then, a child of Congregationalist heritage," Beaumont pronounced. "When I was a boy, I knew a few. I'd say this fella's got a fine pedigree. Doesn't make a damn bit of difference. A malingerer is a malingerer. And yet, the Federalists are a powerful lot with their aristocratic yearnings."

"Set it aside, William. I only told you this as a matter of fact, not to act upon." Thompson held up the jar of bile stones before him and rattled them. "You say these came from one man?"

Beaumont nodded. "Aye. A banker in Plattsburgh. I took care of him for a number of years for gall bladder ailments, and then one evening he took a high fever, turned yellow as a sunflower, and his liver grew tender."

Thompson turned the jar to make them move. "How then?"

"Autopsy."

Thompson set the jar down carefully. "I see. My mother always feared the likes of doctors. Said they would let you succumb to dissect you open."

"It's a belief the profession struggles against. They rioted in Gotham over the doctors taking bodies."

"Truly?"

"Sometime at the end of the last century, more or less. Dr. Chandler, my mentor, he told me about it. It's so hard to persuade the general populace of the value of the autopsy. But you know without it we'd remain as aboriginal root doctors or fall prey to the homoeopaths and other speculative approaches. Draping spiderwebs over wounds. Imagine doing that to the likes of a wound such as Alexis's. Careful inspection of the morbid anatomy is essential for the progress of modern medicine. The French are leaping ahead of us in that regard. There is simply no reason a country as great as ours cannot excel in medicine. Can't you order the lieutenants to testify?"

"William, I can't force them to say what they do not want to say. Besides, what's the worry? Your diagnosis does not depend upon their complaints about Griswold shirking his duty. As you said, scientific facts speak for themselves."

"They do. How then is our malingering Lieutenant Griswold?"

Thompson shook his head slowly. "Reading books and writing in his commonplace book as he awaits his trial."

"Novels I should say."

"Indeed novels. You think it related?"

Beaumont nodded. "I do. The problem with that lovesick trash is that it dissipates a man's resolve and ambition. It's all sentiment without the guide of reason. Like liquor. Deborah reads them for her literary salon. She adores this book *Pamela*. I can understand that habit in women. It's in their nature. But I simply don't understand it in a man. I'd bet lieutenants Russell and Morris read them as well. They're in that salon, you know."

Beaumont shook his head in disbelief. "I do wish you'd talk to those academy men."

AS BEAUMONT WAS WALKING HOME along the hard dirt path between the hospital and his cottage, a man's voice called to him. It was Lieutenant Russell.

"Doctor, do you have a moment, please?"

Beaumont considered the young man. "Not at present, Lieutenant. The hour's late. My wife awaits."

The lieutenant halted some twenty paces away.

"Just a moment, please. Has Major Thompson spoken with you, Doctor?"

"Major Thompson and I speak frequently. How can I help you, Lieutenant?

The lieutenant hesitated.

"Speak, man."

"If I may, Doctor, please, I should like to ask you about Lieutenant Griswold. You see, Doctor, he's a changed man. Whatever it was that ailed him has long left him, and all of us are quite willing to have him back in service. The only consideration that hinders that is your judgment upon Lieutenant Griswold. In light of the facts, might you reconsider?"

"Reconsider?"

"Yes sir. Your report is all that sustains his court-martial."

"Are you suggesting I change the facts? That I lie?"

"No sir, it's just the methods, sir."

"The methods?"

"The methods to ascertain his illness — or whatever it may have been — seemed improper for what we'd expect, like some trick. Unfair and . . ."

Beaumont cut him off.

"Lieutenant Russell, are you in fact suggesting that what I did was somehow wrong?"

The lieutenant hesitated.

"Speak now," Beaumont commanded.

"You're a physician, sir, and the garrison . . ."

"I know what I am, Lieutenant. Get to the point." He pronounced each word like a bullet.

Russell summoned his courage. He raised his voice. "You're a physician, and the garrison looks to you as someone they can trust for help."

Beaumont covered the distance between him and the lieutenant in eleven quick steps. "Mark your speech lest you mar your fortune, young man. Look at me. Look now. By your remark I have every reason to call you out and challenge you right now, sir, right now, for this animadversion upon my honor. Withdraw your remark. Do it now. I said, now."

"Sir, I only meant to say that what you did to Lieutenant Griswold has others worried. I am not questioning your skills as surgeon but appealing to your sentiment of mercy, sir."

"Sentiment of mercy?" Beaumont uttered a sharp laugh. "Lieutenant Russell, I deal in facts. That is what my profession and this fort, this army, expect of me and pay me to do. Lieutenant Griswold is a diagnosed malingerer. That is a fact. Fact, I repeat. Mercy cannot change facts. Leave that to the court or some other authority invested with *that* power. Withdraw your remark now, or choose your weapon. I'm quite serious. Or when we meet next, it shall be on the field of honor."

The lieutenant looked about. The two were entirely alone. He swallowed hard. "Doctor, I withdraw my remark."

Beaumont nodded sharply. "And if I hear one measure of the substance of such remarks pass your or any man's lips on this island, I shall denounce you from one end to the other and call you out with pistols on the field of honor. Am I understood?"

Russell was trembling.

"Yes sir."

{NINE}

THE FIRST FROST CAME ON A CLEAR NIGHT at the end of October with planets visible and stars falling. The surface of the Straits of Mackinac was like glass. A skein of ice formed atop the rain barrels. The last men on the beach gathered round fires in tight circles and coughed from the blue smoke that seemed to follow them even as they shifted and lowered to avoid the smoke.

Six afternoons a week, the women from the literary salon took turns sitting at Alexis's bedside reading to him. They alternated for a month but in time it was Sally Thompson, the major's ailing wife, who took most of the days. Her voice was soft, and she remained wrapped in a shawl as she read. She started with the scriptures, then sonnets, and finally settled on her children's primers. They were all dead now. Alexis enjoyed the primers and would politely interrupt with questions about the characters. He was fascinated by a story about a boy named Peter whose father was a farmer and liked to repeat the phrase that *"Peter had a proper purpose in life."*

By December, the voyageurs' brigades and Indians had long broken up their camps and journeyed into the woods to set their traps. They left behind a beach strewn with debris picked over by dogs and ink-black birds the size of small turkeys with ragged wings whose cries so resembled a plaintive child that the soldiers would discharge their guns into this jetsam. Flocks of geese flew over. Their noise lasted for hours as they passed, casting shadows like clouds.

The island's inhabitants were now reduced to the year-round residents and the soldiers. The season of parties soon began. It was a rotating schedule of teas, salons, dinners and sociables, anything to pass the long, frigid winter days.

In the Crooks's warm parlor, the men stood around the crystal punch bowl filled with a Jamaican rum punch. Deborah sat before the Crooks's latest acquisition, a grand piano. Emilie Crooks sang, her earrings twinkling like stars. It was a song about spring. The Reverend James asked Beaumont if they might talk sometime about the Frenchman. Captain Pearce, close as he was to their exchange, leaned in and suggested they meet at his office. He too wished to hear about the young voyageur with the hole in his side.

The next day they met at the captain's office. Pearce sat behind his desk with his sword upon it. He rubbed the ball of his thumb idly upon the pommel's lion's head. The reverend and Ramsay Crooks sat on the horsehair sofa, and Beaumont eased into a wing chair. A fire hissed with tiny jets of green and yellow flames. They were discussing the Crooks's party. As a corporal poured out cups of coffee, the reverend volunteered that the pleasure of a musical entertainment was the most superior means to pass the winter months. The reverend set down his cup, scratched his arms, cleared his throat.

"Dr. Beaumont, on behalf of the citizens of Mackinac Island, we do commend you for your singular dedication to the care of the voyageur Alexis Martin."

"Thank you, Reverend. It's all in my duty."

The reverend carried on. "We all agree we are most fortunate to have a surgeon of your skill and dedication at this remote garrison. The families of Mackinac Island rest assured."

"Again, thank you, Reverend." Beaumont looked at the assembled company. Ramsay Crooks played with his amethyst ring, his great hips forcing the gaunt reverend into the corner of the small sofa. Captain Pearce, safely planted behind the expanse of his desk, gazed at the frosted window.

The reverend looked as well to these men. But none of them engaged the conversation. He faced Beaumont and once again scratched his arms and cleared his throat.

"We see that the voyageur is largely recovered now. Is that the case?"

"Yes, largely. The orifice into the stomach remains open. But now I'd say he's survived his wounds and is on the way to recovery."

The reverend smiled.

"Excellent. As we all prayed he would be. He did have a difficult healing. I think. We think." The Reverend gestured to Captain Pearce and Crooks. "We think it is proper then to speak of where he shall live. As you know, Doctor, I am the titular magistrate of the borough of Mackinac, and in that capacity I am charged with the civilian affairs of our small government." The reverend hesitated. "Of course in this capacity I consult closely with Captain Pearce and Mister Crooks. Do you have any thoughts on where the lad shall live?" He cocked his head like a dog and waited for an answer.

"Here." Beaumont said simply. "Until he's well enough to travel as he sees fit he should stay here under my care."

"And is he well enough?"

Beaumont considered the question.

"He still needs dressing changes. He still needs to recover his strength. Needs a roof, food, water. So the answer to your question is no."

"We need to make plans."

"Reverend, you are not proposing Alexis St. Martin leave the island?"

"I'm asking whether he's ready to travel as he sees fit."

"Praise for the man's recovery aside, is the purpose of this gathering to tell me Alexis should leave?"

"No, Doctor, we don't want him to leave. We simply want to know whether he is well enough to be discharged from the town's charity roll. Is he?" The reverend's thin eyebrows rose to his question.

"As I say, the wound's not fully healed. Less than three weeks ago it discharged some two tablespoons of pus and material. He still needs dressing changes, still needs to recover his strength, and still can't work. Again, the answer to your question remains a plain no."

The reverend spoke. "Dr. Beaumont, Mackinac Island's charitable coffers are not bottomless. As you well enumerate, he requires room, board, bandages and medications. All those charges have fallen on the town's expense. If he is well enough to travel, it is time for him to continue his care elsewhere. Back in Canada."

"Surely you do not propose to put him in an open bateau and send him off after the ice breaks?"

"With your advice and guidance we propose to outfit him as he needs and send him off. He is rapidly exhausting our charity."

"Immediately?"

"Soon," the reverend replied.

Beaumont looked at Ramsay Crooks.

"Ramsay, he works for the company, does he not? You've got an indenture on him."

"He can't work for the company in his condition. He's not worth a Continental. Mr. Astor himself would discharge me were he to hear we're paying for his upkeep."

The reverend interjected.

"We see the man walking, taking a pipe with some of the soldiers."

Beaumont interrupted the reverend.

"Reverend, the man continues to need treatment. The hole in his side has not healed, and he's still quite debilitated. As I say, there is still foreign material in the wound. A journey in a bateau would likely do him in."

"He's been through worse," Pearce remarked.

Beaumont began to reply. "Are you questioning," he said sharply, but then stopped and took up his coffee cup, but just as quickly he set that down. His hand was trembling.

Pearce folded his arms upon the top of his desk. He considered Beaumont.

"Frankly, Doctor, he's neither soldier nor citizen. I don't doubt you've developed a bit of an attachment to the man, others have as well. I hear some of the ladies have taken to reading to him. Ramsay here even gave him a Bible. But you serve the army and its surgeons' corps. Even if he were a soldier, when he is well enough to travel, he is well enough to leave the service and receive his medical care elsewhere. In Canada. Let the Crown have his bill of fare."

Beaumont began to speak.

"Let me finish please, Doctor. You know the rules. You served in the war, by God, at York, the Niagara frontier, Plattsburgh. I was there too, you know."

Beaumont began to protest, but Pearce cut him off.

"No, Doctor, let me finish. American men with far greater wounds were transported, brave men who took their wounds in combat. You know that. And he's not even one of us."

"Captain, I must insist. I simply must."

Pearce fell silent. Beaumont looked at Crooks, who was gazing into the teepee of his fingers, a smirk cast over his wide face. The reverend sat upright as though tied to a board. His eyes were nearly closed, and his face was entirely without expression.

"Captain," Beaumont said in a measured tone. "That was the war. We did all kinds of things then we'd not hazard now upon any man, friend, foe or pauper. We packed the wounded into a ship's hold so tight that three days later we had to step over the living to gather up the dead to toss into Lake Ontario. We did that because we had no choice. Don't let's bring that into the current consideration."

Pearce thumped his desktop with the ball of his great fist.

"It was the army then," he pronounced. He thumped the desktop again. "It is the army now."

"It was war," Beaumont said plainly. "We behaved differently then. You know it as well as I do. We had our mission. Our orders."

Pearce raised his chin, all the while looking at Beaumont. Then he looked away, at the window, the fire, the floor.

"Doctor," he said quietly, "I think I speak not only for the army as the commander of this garrison but for the company, as well as the civil government, when I say that neither borough nor garrison nor company can be home to many more men like Edgar and Alexis. The hospital is a hospital. Not a boardinghouse for your charity cases."

"Here, here," said Crooks. "'Tis the heart of the matter, is it not, Reverend?"

The reverend kept his eyes closed.

"And Edgar has value. Look at the work he does," Beaumont insisted.

Crooks chuckled. "But an illiterate French Canadian fur trapper with a hole in his side has little prospects for advancement. Except perhaps in a circus."

"He can do chores as well as any man, Ramsay."

Crooks raised his thick eyebrows.

"Well then, perhaps that indenture is not wholly lost? He could do some chores for the company. We might well have a place for a simple laborer."

Reverend James lifted his thin eyelids like some china doll set upright and made his appeal.

"Then, Doctor, he is ready to leave the island."

"Reverend, Ramsay, I meant that in time he can do that. In time."

"How much time, Doctor?" the reverend asked.

"It is hard to say."

"And yet you say he's recovered."

"Gentlemen, where is mercy?" Beaumont appealed. "He's an innocent man. The victim of bad fortune."

Ramsay Crooks chuckled.

Beaumont ignored him.

"Do you gentlemen think that the island's inhabitants shall wish to be party to such a cold decision?" He looked at Reverend James. "Reverend, by this act, all the charity rendered is undone."

The reverend puckered his lips.

"Dr. Beaumont, please, I think I speak for the island's inhabitants when I say let's not contest either the depth or the sincerity of our charity. We're Christians, and we're Americans. Beneficence is an obligation, but it is, I submit, a limited obligation. One man cannot be an insatiable draw upon the charity of the borough. We have other commitments to charity, the mission school, for instance. I personally place great pride in our efforts to give the Indian children a Christian education. Think of the potential that is to come from that investment. That one day our red brethren might rise in the scale of social civilization when Education and Christianity should go hand in hand to make the wilderness blossom as the rose."

Beaumont pleaded.

"Reverend, let us not balance the life of one invalid against those of a schoolroom of children."

The reverend was unusually animated. "Doctor, I do not intend to even suggest that the one is traded for the other. Let me remind you that in the days of the British occupation, I've every expectation your Frenchman would have been carried out on a board long before the first freeze and buried in the bone orchard. I know I speak for the town that we have made our fair charitable contribution. We wish our denizens to be useful. We defer of course to your medical judgment, but we see the man able and well enough to walk about, to eat and drink. He seems well enough to travel as soon as the weather permits."

Beaumont began to speak, but the captain cut him off.

"Neither the island's inhabitants nor the Great Lakes command shall be drawn into this issue. Understood?"

Beaumont was perplexed.

"Shall not be drawn in with circulars or pamphlets or other public pronouncements about the fate of some Gumbo fur trapper with a hole in his side. No letters to generals. Do I make myself clear, Doctor?"

Beaumont hesitated.

"Yes. Yes, Captain Pearce, you do."

IN THE DAYS FOLLOWING THE MEETING at the captain's office, Beaumont felt like he was back in the company store on the day of the shooting, when Crooks and Pearce had him cornered, except this time he could not free himself of Crooks's grip. All the triumph and joy of the last seven months of caring for Alexis were fast disappearing. In their place was a growing despair.

For days, Beaumont spoke not a word of the meeting as he tried to go about his business. He needed time to think of a plan. It was after dinner one day that Beaumont decided finally to tell Deborah about the decision to send Alexis away. They were seated at their kitchen table, their dishes set to one side. They had been talking about Sarah. The child was nearly walking, quick bouncing steps, her arms outstretched like some flightless bird. Now they sat in the peace of each other's quiet, listening to the sound of the winter evening about their cottage. The skitter of a small animal passed beneath the floor.

"There's been some news about Alexis," he said.

He told her how the town, the company and the village were united in their conviction that Alexis had exhausted their charity. "They just want him to go," he concluded. "But he's not ready."

"Why?"

"Because they fear he shall be a pauper. They say he's drained or will drain the town's charity, that there are no more funds to support his care. The Presbyterian Board of Missions is more dedicated to the school than to the invalid."

"That's terrible. I've worried something was wrong. You've been so quiet of late."

He looked at her. "What do you think of him staying here until he's healed?"

"Here with us?"

"Yes Deb, here. Just for a while. He can stay in the back room."

She looked about the room. "Move him here?"

"Yes."

"Until the boat is ready to take him away? Why can he not just stay in the hospital as he is and then depart when he is well?"

"He'll stay there as long as he can, but come spring, after the ice breaks, they'll surely want him gone. When that happens, we could take him in here."

"I thought you had no desire to make him your charity case?"

"Circumstances alter cases."

"Such as?"

"His is a complex case, and it's not done."

"Is he well enough to travel?"

"No, not yet. You've seen yourself how he still needs my care. And even if he is well enough to travel, I cannot in good professional conscience simply submit to the town's callous will and see him off a pauper in a bateau where in time he will surely succumb. I cannot tolerate an act of callous folly that involves my patient. It's what they ordered us to do at York. Pack the wounded men in boats and then set sail. Men died in that ship."

"But here with us?" She closed her eyes.

"He'll just sleep here. During the day the room shall be free and you can continue to use it and . . ."

"And what will he do during the day?"

Beaumont was startled. It was not like Deborah to interrupt.

"The chores of a common servant," he explained. "If he can, if he's well enough. Chop wood, haul slops and trash, sweep out the kitchen, bank the fire, carry the ashes from the fireplace. I'd like to have the bushes cut back to make more room for Sarah to play. Soon she'll be running. The roof needs mending too."

"William, I don't question your professional judgment. I don't. And yet, if the man is well enough to do those many tasks of an able-bodied man, well then, I for one cannot see why he is not well enough to travel back to Lower Canada."

"His dressings need changing. They're quite complicated."

"But he won't travel alone," she said. "I remember in the war how they moved men with all kinds of wounds. And it wasn't always in a ship's hold. Surely they'll send him with others making the journey. After the thaw, boats come in and out of the harbor regularly. If Elias Farnham can change the bandages, well then, others can learn too. It strikes me as simple as sewing. I've seen it done myself when I've read to him at the hospital."

"Deborah," he nearly begged.

"William, you can be so single-minded. Yes, he's your patient, but what about us? Your family? It's hard enough as it is living on this island. Besides, what of the funds to care for him and to feed him? Our monies are tight. Have you thought how we shall support him as well as our children?"

"Children?" His eyes widened.

She nodded.

"Deborah, are you with child?"

"I hadn't wanted to tell you yet, and I should talk with Helen, for this has happened before and meant nothing. It's that feeling in the morning I can relieve with breakfast. But there's no quickening. Still, even if I'm not pregnant, the point still remains, William. You need to think of our family. You work so hard, and yet our funds are limited."

He reached across the table for her hand. Their fingers entwined. He leaned over and kissed her palm, and held her hand between his.

"Deborah, my love, please don't say that."

"Then make the choice that is right for *us,*" she insisted. "If he's well enough to do chores, he can do chores for the company. They have ample money. We don't. You've done quite enough for the man, and you're a hero for that. Surely others can see fit to do their part?"

"But if the others don't?"

She gazed at her husband. She smiled. "Perhaps I say this because it's a woman's custom to submit to some higher will. There's control and then there is the illusion of that control. And sometimes you men can be so charmed by that illusion. Why don't we just fret over what the others do, or don't do, when we have to?"

TEN

THROUGHOUT THE WINTER ALEXIS CONTINUED his slow recovery. Some days, after Beaumont awakened him for the morning dressing change, he would gulp spoonfuls of broth and bites of bread and then collapse back onto his cot and sleep for hours, rising only to relieve himself in a chamber pot. On good afternoons, he walked back and forth across the hospital floor with the aid of his cane, counting off the number of turns he took. Then he began to walk without the cane. Beaumont brought him a new pair of boots and a pair of woolen stockings that Deborah had knitted. By February, Alexis was able to take slow walks in the snow.

Though the wound still extruded occasional bits of matter, his injuries, with the exception of the hole into his stomach, were firmly scarred. The hole had changed little since the sixth week after the shooting. It was some two and a half inches around, and food and drink constantly exuded unless prevented by a tent of lint, soft compress and elastic bandage. The wound was nearly painless except for a thin rim of tissue between the muscles of the ribs and the coat of the stomach that was as sensitive to the touch of a fingertip or instrument as a blistered surface.

Over the course of the winter, the routine of the dressing changes began to change. Some mornings, when the demands of Beaumont's other patients were light and he had time to spare before he dressed the wound, he would have Alexis lie flat upon his cot so that he could dangle a piece of meat into the cavity by means of a silken thread. Beaumont used a quarter-hour sandglass to measure the time it took for the flesh to dissolve. Alexis's noon meal became a source of occasional study as well. If Beaumont was present at the start of the meal and had a free hour, he would wait until Alexis finished eating, then undo Alexis's dressings to insert a siphon. He would draw off some of the gastric contents in intervals to inspect the pace and appearance of digestion, or he would just sit upon a stool and gaze into the hole.

What most fascinated Beaumont was the clear fluid he came to call the "gastric liquor." Beaumont had observed that if the hole was not properly dressed, the stomach, when it was entirely empty and contracted upon itself, would extrude itself out through the aperture like a hen's egg. When he touched this tissue with the tip of his finger, it grew tumescent papilla and emitted a clear liquid that felt like water. Its taste was astringent. He tried positioning a cup to gather the liquid, but the process was slow, the yield trivial, and Alexis soon grew irritated and insisted on shifting his position.

In time, an idea came to him like a thunderclap. One afternoon at the company store, he had seen Theodore Mathews's daughter use a gum elastic tube to suck up a glass of honeyed tea until she drained the glass, her lips pursed and cheeks sunken.

The length of tube cost three cents.

He tried it out the next morning, when Alexis's stomach was entirely empty. He positioned Alexis on his right side so that the stomach gently collapsed inward into its natural state, and then he inserted the thin length of gum elastic tube some five inches into the cavity. Alexis winced as the tube brushed against the tender margin of the hole.

"Now roll onto your left side," Beaumont commanded.

Alexis hesitated.

"Left," Beaumont repeated.

"*Gauche,*" Alexis muttered, and he turned as Beaumont, his hands gripping his patient's thin waist, positioned the orifice in a dependent location. The end of the tube stuck out like a queer straw.

In just a few seconds, the clear liquor began flowing from the end of the tube. At first single drops, but in time it was a steady dribble. Beaumont collected these drops into a glass vial he held beneath the end of the tube. Alexis moaned.

"Doctor, I'm sick."

"Tell me." Beaumont's gaze was intent on the vial.

His voice was a measured calm. *Aequanimitas,* he thought. He continued to move the tube. More drops flowed.

"There." Alexis whimpered as he breathed heavily. "In the pit. What's wrong with me?"

Beaumont continued moving the tube.

"It's dark now, Doctor."

The drops of clear liquor continued to flow. Beaumont held the tube steady.

"Doctor, please." Alexis begged.

"You feel faint?" Beaumont asked steadily.

Alexis swallowed hard. "Like I'm drunk. But I have not drunk in days. What's wrong?"

"I know, Alexis. You'll be fine. Just rest."

He stroked the lad's side as he collected a few more drops, and then he slipped the tube out. He lay it carefully upon the tabletop and took up the cork, sealed the vial firmly and held it upward, thumb on the bottom and forefinger on the top, so that the light flowing in through the small window illuminated the vial. There was perhaps one ounce. He gently agitated the contents. It was beautiful, entirely clear, without a trace of sediment, little if any viscosity.

Alexis was staring at it as well. "What is that?" he whispered.

"Gastric liquor," Beaumont pronounced. "Pure gastric liquor."

"Liquor? But I have not drunk."

"I know. It's in there. You made it, so to speak."

"Did you drain it all?"

"No. Not all."

Alexis exhaled slowly.

"And it hurt so, like I was to vomit. Next time just take it all out."

Beaumont slipped the vial into the small pocket of his vest. "We'll see. Now let's get this wound dressed and get you some breakfast."

Brief though the experiment was, the result was incontrovertible, and he was ecstatic. He could gather the liquor, study it and, ultimately, discover what this clear fluid was.

BY APRIL, the daytime temperature rose above freezing sufficient to melt the snow. The pathways among the barracks, hospital, houses and company buildings soon became a slurry of liver-colored mud. In the evening the pathways would freeze so that come morning, lines of soldiers set forth like blue ants to spread sand and sawdust. They laid out boards, and these narrow paths afforded easy travel to and from the barracks, village and company buildings. Men began to laugh again, and Edgar was heard singing.

One weekend the ice vanished from the straits, almost as abruptly as it had formed some six months before. The winter storms and the retreat of the ice swept away the debris the previous occupants had left upon the beach. A crew set out with fresh-cut logs to repair the corduroy road that led up from the harbor to Market Street and then on to the fort. Overnight, the land turned green, the air smelled of soil and the buds of the rhododendron swelled as thick as a great toe. Mackinac was ready for another season of commerce.

Before the month was over, the first of the resupply ships arrived from Detroit. Beaumont watched from a bench near the dockyard as the soldiers and company men celebrated the new bull to replace the one they had slaughtered last fall. There were cages of chickens, seven squealing piglets, sacks of flour and meal, crates of dry goods, barrels of wines and rattling crates of brandies and Madeira, and to the delight of several of the men and boys, wheels of cheese. Mathews chuckled at the inventory of the winter's consumption of some thirty gallons Tenerifte wine, four and a half gallons port wine, ten gallons best Madeira, seventy gallons red wine and nine gallons brandy.

Within days, the voyageurs' and Indians' boats appeared on the horizon. Some afternoons when Beaumont and Major Thompson leaned upon the parapet of Fort Hill to witness the traffic upon the waters, they counted at least fifty bateaux and canoes laden with pelts and buffalo robes. The beach was once again a crowded field of wigwams, wickiups and tents. The barking of dogs, the shouts and screams of little brown children and the chatter of men and women at their cooking fires created a constant din. In the evenings, the fires were like a reflection of the night sky, their clusterings denoting the alliances of their creators in this cosmopolis of trade. Ramsay Crooks was pleased with the value of this season's haul.

"It must have been a brutal cold on the plain, brutal cold," he announced as he inspected the thick nap of a buffalo robe some seven feet long. "And have you seen the ermine pelts, have you ever seen such a virginal white? And so soft. Brings tears to my eyes."

He rubbed a pelt against his cheek.

Under the dispassionate regard of Captain Pearce and Major Thompson, Theodore Mathews, armed with clipboard and carbon pencil, directed the company clerks as they hauled from the warehouses crates full of trinkets and goods for trade. These they set out on tables fashioned from boards set across crates and barrels.

Mathews, with his habit for order, arranged the trade goods alphabetically. There were rolls of blankets, broad cord, gray cloth, boxes and crates full of boxwood combs, biscuit, brass jewsharps, beaver shot, common needles and darning needles, cotton bandanna handkerchiefs, ivory combs, ingrain worsted thread, ink powder, japanned quart jacks, kettle chains, *maitre de rels,* men's shirts, men's imitation beaver hats, moon paper, nun's thread, nails, northwest guns, plain bath rings, pierced brooches, scalping knives, St. Lawrence shells, stone rings, sturgeon twine, stitching thread, snuff, snuff boxes, snaffle bridles, stirrup irons, tomahawks and tobacco. And most cherished, and thus guarded by a pair of soldiers, small barrels of whiskey. Within days the boxes and crates of goods were replaced four times, the warehouses filled with furs. The company store was crowded from dawn to dusk.

Week after week, spring into summer, they would carry on like this. Theodore Mathews delivered the day's neatly printed receipts to the office, where Ramsay Crooks and his eldest son worked diligently and quietly over their accounts. The company men and the soldiers paced the parapets of Fort Hill, smoked and swapped stories as they waited for the next wave of traders to arrive. The Reverend James and his wife taught scripture to one dozen Indian children at the mission school.

"What do they do with the carcasses?" Beaumont asked Major Thompson one afternoon as they gazed down upon the bedlam of trade from the heights of the fort.

"They?"

"The trappers. What do they do with the carcasses of the buffalo and such? Eat them?"

The major shrugged. "Perhaps some. Or leave them where they skinned them."

"There must be piles of bones out there."

The major nodded. "Perhaps the next great industry," he observed.

"And then what?"

{ELEVEN}

IN JUNE, ONE YEAR AFTER THE SHOOTING, a corporal delivered a note to Beaumont. It was the bill for last month's expenses for Alexis's room and board. As Beaumont read it, his temples pounded. The borough had returned this bill to the army without remittance, and over it Captain Pearce had scrawled in a jagged script:

William,
Gone by July.
Capt Isaiah Ignatius Pearce

He wadded up the note and tossed it to the floor. He slapped his desktop.

"Alexis is my patient, *mine,* not theirs. They think they have me cornered," he murmured. "I'll fight them with charity."

Two days later, on a clear Saturday afternoon, the Beaumont family sat in their sitting room. Sarah was absorbed with a doll. Deborah had paused her reading of a favorite passage from *Pamela* to gaze at Sarah and then at a window pot of geraniums that had just bloomed. She was smiling. Beaumont was at the table with his leather notebook opened before him. He had finished tabulating the balance of their household accounts and savings. This winter's fees were numerous. Their accounts were, finally, truly whole. In the past two years he had earned some $250 from the Office of Indian Affairs vaccinating the Indians against the pox. The results inspired confidence. He set down his carbon pencil and asked if he might talk with Deborah about Alexis.

She closed the book over her thumb to mark her place. "Of course."

"I'd like to move him here to stay in the back room."

She set her book down beside her. "So the town has not rescinded its decision?"

"Of course not. Money overflows the place, but not one cent for charity."

"Well then, why can't he leave?"

"Deborah please, let me explain."

"Go ahead," she said plainly.

"Perhaps he's well enough to travel. But you've seen for yourself that he still needs my care. He can't leave with that wound as it is because it's not yet healed. There is still a passage directly into his stomach, and as long as it is open, whatever he eats or drinks simply passes out like a stoved-in tap at the bottom of a barrel. Unless of course it's dressed, and then all's well. The stomach works as well as any man's. You see how he has gained his strength, and he walks about now, but as long as that wound remains open he has a direct passage from his stomach to open air."

Beaumont stopped speaking. "Do you gather what I mean? Are you listening to me? Deborah?"

She sat mutely with her hands folded upon her lap. She was looking at Sarah.

"Deborah, look at me please? Could you grant your husband that simple courtesy?"

She raised her eyes.

"Don't you see, Deborah, that to send him off now while he's healthy but still wounded is like throwing a pearl into the lake? He will heal."

"What do you mean a pearl, William?"

"He's a singular case. Singular. True, my library's limited, but I cannot find a case like his."

He was pacing. Sarah squatted upon her chubby thighs, her tiny heels tucked into her swaddled crotch, her doll idle in her lap. She looked up wide-eyed at her father as he passed back and forth, back and forth before her.

"I can't just let him leave. And if he does and he ends up in another physician's care, most surely I'll hear that physician's laughter clear across Lake Huron at the folly of the man who sent this prize off in a bateau because the citizens of the town could not muster a few dollars a month to keep him fed, housed and bandaged."

"Prize? William, what do you mean? He's your patient."

"Of course he is. Don't you see, Deborah, that the case is not yet done? There's an opportunity here that I simply cannot ignore. When he heals, I will write it up. I've taken careful notes since the day of the shooting. It just needs to be completed, and once it is complete, I shall send it to the *Medical Recorder*. This is a once-in-a-lifetime opportunity. I have every reason to expect the recognition for my efforts will be substantial. I have every expectation that Surgeon General Lovell will see this as reason for my promotion to surgeon.

"Deborah, listen to me, please. When he lies on his side, I can look directly into the cavity and see the process of digestion. I've seen things no other physician has. Seen beef digested. I've seen wonderful things. And I saved his life. Don't you see? If he leaves now, what sort of ending is that to the case report? That we cast him off in a boat to travel some one thousand miles and fend for himself? A case worthy of the *Medical Recorder* cannot conclude like that."

She gazed down at her novel. "I don't read such reports."

"But you know what a good story is. That you do. This cannot end like some tragedy of Shakespeare. It requires a good ending."

"When, how, will it end?"

"I beg you, Deborah, just to give me time. I need time for him to heal. He needs to heal, and when he is healed, the case is done and my paper is done."

"He stays in the back room then? Will he eat with us?"

Beaumont considered her question. "We can't expect him to pay his way when he has nothing. Besides, he'll work for us. It will help build his character."

Deborah shook her head. "I meant, will we share table with him? He's a nice enough young man, but he's a bit queer."

She stopped speaking. But he said nothing.

"William, don't you see? I'm not in the army. I live here on an island with just eight women I can talk with. I have to suffer Emilie Crooks for the use of her piano, no letters for the months of winter. We shall have another child in the winter. And now you propose to bring an invalid voyageur into our house."

She held a handkerchief at her mouth.

"Deborah, I know life here is difficult. I know that. It is for me as well. And that's precisely why we need to help Alexis. My career has always been only halfway to what I want, to what I deserve. When I first enlisted in the army, during the war, it was to be as a surgeon or even an assistant surgeon. But they made me a mere surgeon's mate. When the fighting ended, I deserved promotion to assistant surgeon, and yet, despite all my labors and successes, they would only offer me my same commission as a mate. At York, I operated side by side with the surgeons, just as one of them. When other doctors fled the army, I remained, even in the winter, along the Niagara frontier. When Plattsburgh was under siege and half the town fled and begged that we sue the British for peace, I joined in the fighting. I dodged bullets at Fort Moreau to tend to the wounded. I've a letter signed by General Macomb and seventeen other officers that testifies of my bravery in that battle. But eight years later, after hard work in private practice, when I sought to reenlist, they would not grant me commission as a surgeon, but only as an assistant surgeon. And do you know why I have suffered these repeated indignities upon my talent and my character?"

She shook her head slowly. "No," she whispered.

"Because I, a New England farmer's son who set out in this world with little more than my wits and my ambition, I was trained not in a medical college, but as an apprentice bound by an indenture, much like these voyageurs who gather beaver pelts for Ramsay Crooks. That has vexed my career since the day the Third Medical Society of Vermont granted me a license. That training has been my blessing, and it has been my curse. But here, with this case, I finally have something to show, and show definitively, my talents as a surgeon and a physician.

"I saved his life. I nurtured him to health. And now, if I can close the wound, I will have managed entirely on my own an unprecedented case. When Dr. Lovell reads this account of the wound he will surely see the rightness of my promotion, and when colleagues read the case, they will surely grant me the recognition due to me. Now and forever. The circumstances of my training will be of no consideration in the judgment of my character and the merit of my skill. This is America, not some aristocracy. A man is judged for what he has achieved, not from whence he came."

He stopped speaking abruptly. A sob welled within his chest.

Deborah stared at her husband.

"I had never known of this, William," she whispered.

Beaumont composed himself.

"I know," he said. "I always thought I should not burden you with something I felt unable to change, until now. Because now I can change it."

"By your accounts do we have the money for this?"

"We can cover his expenses, yes. I see no reason to pay him for his work. That'll be fair compensation for his care, room and board. In time, Deborah, with this investment and my promotion to surgeon, we'll have the money we need for our house and land."

"What does he say?"

"Say?"

"About this plan?"

"I should expect he'd be grateful for our charity. When you consider his wound and his poverty, what choice does he have?"

She looked around their small and crowded room. "Yes, what choice." She nodded. "When does he move in?"

"I'm not sure, but I'd hazard any day now. Pearce returned his bills to me and wrote that he wants him gone by July. But of course, who we take into our house is a private matter."

She lowered her eyes. "As you wish. We'll need a place for the child by the winter. We could perhaps move Sarah here to the front room. But enough. I don't want to talk any more about this. I trust you."

He took Sarah into his arms and stepped closer to Deborah.

"Please don't despair. It was luck that brought us together, and now much good will come. He will continue to heal, and in time I'll have the recognition I require for promotion."

"How much time?"

"Time?" He considered her question. "That, Deborah, I just don't know. A few months, perhaps. Perhaps more."

{TWELVE}

ON JULY 1, 1823, ALEXIS ST. MARTIN was settled into the slope-roofed back room of the Beaumont household. Convincing Alexis to accept this plan proved easy. After Beaumont explained it to Alexis, Alexis stammered in a confused garble of French and English. Beaumont heard words like "home" and "Canada." He raised his hand as if to signal a halt. Alexis swallowed.

"And who will care for your wound?"

Alexis gazed at his bandaged torso.

"Who?" Beaumont insisted.

Alexis shrugged. Beaumont sat beside him.

"Be sensible, Alexis. You know what I have done for you for many months, and am still wishing to do for you to see that healed. But you can't remain in this hospital. Ramsay Crooks and his people, the town, they won't permit it."

Beaumont reached out and placed the length of his right arm upon Alexis's shoulders.

"Trust me, Alexis. I know what it's like to be alone in the world with little prospect for advancement. I know what it's like to be hungry, to fret whether you can afford even a crust. When I was a young man, about your age, Dr. Chandler took me in as an apprentice. In three years time, I'd grown up and gained a valuable skill. Now I'm older and you're here and you need help, and I want to help you."

"You were shot too?"

"No, no, I was well, but like you I had little more than debts." He took a deep breath. "Alexis, you're like a son to me. I, we—my wife and I—we'll take good care of you."

The young man nodded.

In time, the days' routines developed. They began just after sunrise with Beaumont changing Alexis's dressings as Deborah prepared breakfast. Alexis would splash water over his face from a bucket he kept in his room, run water through his hair, comb it with his fingers and dress in knee breeches and an old flannel shirt of Beaumont's that fit him like a smock. He set to his chores, restocking the woodbin, all the while whistling, then took his seat, arms crossed upon the tabletop, his hair shiny black and pulled back flat over his skull. He ate quickly, using only a knife and his fingers, smacking his lips, tipping his bowl to drink whatever liquid remained. He licked his knife, wiped the plate clean with a thick slice of bread or boiled potato he'd saved for the task.

As Alexis ate, Deborah straightened the house and set away the previous evening's dishes, and Beaumont sat at his worktable reviewing his visitation log as he drank his coffee. The infant Sarah clung to her mother's skirts, staring wide-eyed at the new man in the house. While the Beaumonts ate, Alexis would carry in pails of water from the well to refill the pitchers, carry out the breakfast scraps, his oddly wide feet slapping upon the hearthstones. After the meal, he scoured the dishes.

He occupied the remainder of the day with routine chores, a nap and an afternoon walk about the garrison and village. He was clever at some simple tasks, scraping out the ashes while still keeping the cooking fire kindled, scrubbing a pot, sweeping a floor and carrying the waste out on a shingle. He was handy not only with whittling but with wood chopping as well, and within weeks had set to splitting rounds of wood with a slow determination. It became his habit to see Beaumont off to the hospital and then walk out to the side of the Beaumonts' cottage with ax, mallet and wedge and set to work upon the logs.

Deborah kept him out of the sitting room, and in all his time in Mackinac he never once, at least to her knowledge, entered their bedroom. Their kitchen, his slope-roofed back room and the yard were the extent of his domain. In time, his range extended to the island and the camps along the beach as well.

ONE AFTERNOON, as Deborah dandled Sarah upon her knee while Alexis swept out the kitchen, she told Alexis that he needed a haircut. He stopped his sweeping, folded his hands atop the broom handle and smiled at her. She held her fore and middle fingers into a V shape and ran them scissor wise through her own hair.

"Haircut," she repeated. "It's gotten rather long." She held a lock of her own hair out to demonstrate.

"Yes, yes," he nodded, as he pushed back his black locks from his face. "A haircut."

Within the hour she had him outdoors seated on a chair beneath a shade tree, a gray sheet wrapped around him like a high-collared dress, his black locks falling as she worked her shears. Sarah sat before them constructing piles with stacks of short straight sticks he had whittled smooth for her to play with, and Rex lay upon his side, his thick tail thumping the ground.

In the evenings, after Alexis returned from his afternoon wanderings, he would find Deborah preparing the evening meal, and he would attend to

Sarah as her mother cooked. He had by now accumulated a small set of carvings of various creatures that he amused Sarah with. He sang her songs in French. Supper done, Deborah would serve Alexis alone as she read to him from the Bible while waiting for Beaumont to return from his patients.

"You read different books," he said to her. "Not the one Madame Sally read."

"It is the best book," she said. "Swallow a bit before you speak, Alexis."

He looked confused.

She indicated her mouth.

"Don't speak with a mouth full of food."

He looked at his plate, then looked at Deborah. He was blushing.

At the pace he ate, the reading would end within ten minutes.

The summer grew unusually hot. By August, the heat was so intense and unremitting it drove families to sleep outdoors beneath canopies of bug netting. Work slowed, and people lingered under the trees along the lakeshore, fanning themselves. The women wrapped their skirts about their hips and waded into the lake and splashed water over their heads. Some gave up all pretension and walked out into the lake far enough that their skirts rose up about them as though their torsos were at the center of great blossoms. Some men simply sat in the water. Others wandered out as deep as their shoulders. Ramsay Crooks was seen floating upon his back, a great berg dressed in trousers and a cotton blouse.

Alexis regularly walked with Rex trotting beside. He had befriended several of the clerks, voyageurs and Indians who gathered about the shacks and outer buildings surrounding the dock. The men passed long hours lying in the afternoon shade, and at night, they sat around fires on the beach. They roasted what meat they could purchase or trade for. They drank anything that came from a bottle. By the close of summer, people began talking of the man with the hole in his side and his appetite for whiskey and song and his talent with a carving knife. Rumors began to circulate of his complicity in acts of petty vandalism, his instigation of fights. Deborah begged her husband to discipline him.

HAVING ALEXIS IN THE HOUSE afforded Beaumont easy access to observe the process of digestion. Within a month, Beaumont began more frequent and sometimes extended periods of observation and careful note taking. These required removing and reapplying new bandages to keep the stomach contents from spilling out. Alexis was ordered to lie without even shifting. He became a living cadaver.

The rigors of these observations and the failure of the wound to close began to frustrate Alexis. One long summer afternoon, as Beaumont was observing the effect of the gastric digestion on a piece of raw beef he'd dangled into the cavity by means of a silk string, Alexis reached down and began to pull at the thread. Beaumont swept Alexis's hand away.

"Alexis, stop that!" he ordered. "What are you doing?"

Alexis' face was twisted with anger. "*Putain, ça craint! Suffit!* That's enough," he cried. "Enough! This is not working. Whatever it is you try to do to me, it is not working."

Beaumont stared at Alexis.

"When will I be healed?" Alexis demanded.

"Healed?"

"Closed up for good so I can go. Go," he yelled. "As you promised."

"Calm down, Alexis. It's healing slowly, boy. You have to be patient."

Alexis stared at Beaumont. His pupils were dilated, and his lips quivered. "It was a year." He began speaking, but then he stopped.

The two men stared at each other.

"You've got to be patient."

"Why's it not closed?"

"Honestly, Alexis, these sorts of wounds take time. Trust me. I took care of such things in the war. You're fortunate to be alive. Be patient."

"Why's it not closed?" Alexis insisted.

Beaumont straightened his frame. "Why? I don't know why. But if you insist, well then, I could try sewing it closed."

"Try?"

"With a needle. Sew it closed." Beaumont mimicked the action of sewing.

Alexis considered the idea.

"Now?"

"No, not immediately, but after your meal digests."

Alexis grabbed a wad of bandages and held it over the hole. He straightened himself up upon the edge of his cot.

"Why didn't you do that before?"

"Before?"

"Why have you waited to sew it up?"

Beaumont's eyes narrowed. "I have not *waited,* Alexis. I've thought it wise to let Nature take its course of healing. But if you insist, I can try to sew it up. It will require several stitches to bring the margins together, sort of like a purse. Of course, I can guarantee nothing. But if you insist."

He made to raise his hand to once again mimic the act of stitching, but it was trembling, and so he clasped his hands together as if he was kneading something small and pliant.

"Will it hurt?" Alexis asked.

Beaumont snorted a laugh. "Of course."

Alexis slapped his bed frame. "Why didn't you sew it closed when it first happened?"

Beaumont regarded Alexis.

"Are you, are you *actually* questioning my medical methods? Is that what you're doing, after all I have done for you, now, to have this conversation here, here in my house?"

Alexis lowered his eyes.

"No *docteur,* no sir."

"I'll see fit to sew the wound up, when the wound is fit for sewing up. My prescribed treatment is to let Nature follow its course of healing by my careful ministrations, and that has done quite well for you. Now be a good patient, and please lie back." Beaumont patted the surface of the mattress. "And while we're on this matter of your healing, let me assure you that intoxication will not aid in your healing."

Alexis looked confused.

"Drinking to the point of silliness, Alexis, will not aid in closing up that hole. If you fail to maintain a robust constitution, that hole won't close up. Moreover, think of your reputation and mine as well. It upsets Mrs. Beaumont. She thinks of you as a son, as do I."

Alexis gazed at his doctor. "I'm sorry," he mumbled, and then he slowly lowered himself upon his back.

⁘{THIRTEEN}⁘

THE FIRST WEEKS OF SEPTEMBER BEGAN with drenching rains that carved rivulets into the roads followed by days so warm that men walked about at noon in their shirtsleeves. The Reverend James's roses produced a new set of blooms, and women sweated before their kitchen fires. Still, the soldiers and company men set to repairing the island's rickety buildings and packing the storehouses with supplies. The pause in these labors came with the autumn dance.

The Beaumonts and Sally and Hardage Thompson left the dance before nightfall. Deborah's pregnancy exhausted her. As the four of them were making their way home along the path, Beaumont spied Alexis in the company of a group of voyageurs. He excused himself from his wife and friends and called Alexis over to him.

"Allo, Doctor," Alexis sang. He was swaying and grinning with drink. His hair was matted with sweat, and he was dressed like the other voyageurs in a kind of loose white pantaloons and a red kerchief about his neck. Beaumont reached out and set his hands upon the young man's shoulders. His breath smelled of liquor.

"Alexis, take care tonight. People are watching you, watching us. Please? Remember what I said about reputation."

"But of course," he laughed. "We are like dishes. Easily cracked." And then he loped off into the night.

SEVERAL HOURS LATER, a hard knocking upon the front door roused Beaumont from his shallow sleep. Deborah stirred, but she did not awaken. He slipped out from under the quilt, stepped past his daughter's crib and felt his way blindly to the front door. He opened it to face the silhouettes of two men, their uniforms visible in sharp silhouette. He leaned with one arm against the frame and kept his other arm crooked over his brow to shield his eyes against the glare of their lantern.

"Lower that, can you not?"

"Pardon, Doctor." The man holding the lantern set it upon the ground. The circle of light shimmered and settled.

Beaumont looked at the men, squinting. "What is it?"

THE TAKER MADE MAD

"Cap'n Pearce sent us, sir. There's been a stabbing. One of the voyageurs is cut up bad."

Beaumont looked back into the darkness of his small house. Nothing was visible save the glow of the kitchen coals and the exaggerated shadows of the iron cooking wares suspended above that feeble light.

"Alexis?" he asked the darkness.

"I don't know, sir, but you'd best come quick. We've laid him out in one of the warehouses. He bleeds heavy despite bandages."

"Give me a minute to dress, and one of you fetch Elias Farnham. I've a lantern here I can use." He turned back to the soldiers. "Go then now!"

BEAUMONT FOUND THE WOUNDED MAN laid out on a cot with his head turned aside to better accommodate a cabbage-sized wad of bloody dressings that covered the wound. He recognized the voyageur from the St. Louis brigade. The man spoke little English, and the bits he did speak were incomprehensible.

Elias Farnham arrived, and he and Beaumont set to work peeling away the bandages. The man's lips were pale and his skin the color of old flour. The wound described a clean downward cutting motion along the length of his neck, angled from the back of his left ear to the tip of the collarbone, engaging the strap muscles, several veins and a knick to an artery that sprayed a small fountain of blood. Blood ran over the man's cheek, through his hair, over his chest and down the back of his neck. In time, they discovered another wound. A clean slash into the abdomen.

Beaumont and Farnham worked on the man for over an hour, stitching and packing the wounds, until they had his abdomen and the whole of his neck and head, with apertures for his mouth and nose, wrapped in gauze dressings. The area around the neck was stained a crimson gorgelet.

It was when they were washing their instruments and scraping the blood from beneath their fingernails, that the sound of boots came heavy upon the floor. Captain Pearce stood at the foot of the cot. He still wore his dress uniform from that evening's dance. He rested his right hand on the pommel of his sword.

"Well?"

"The man's lost a lot of blood. A lot. Still, I've managed to staunch most of the bleeding. The wound to the abdomen may have nicked bowel."

Pearce swayed a bit at his place where he stood. "Has he said anything? Said who did it?"

Beaumont shook his head. "Nothing sensible."

He looked to Elias, who shook his head as well.

Pearce let out a kind of indignant snort. "I got a couple of Blackfeathers under arrest. One of 'em's your Frenchman. Your patient. And Edgar too. Seems that all the island's finest society came out in full fig for the Gumbo ball."

Pearce shook his head slowly.

Beaumont set down the forceps he was washing. "Captain?"

"Facts are that your boy was the object of a disputation which led to this fight between the Blackfeathers and the St. Louis brigades. So I'm having him and a couple of his comrades sober up in the brig, and we'll see what he says in the morning."

He touched two fingers to the brim of his hat.

"My greetings to Mrs. Beaumont. We missed the two of you at the dance, but I understand she's soon to be lying in with child." Pearce turned to leave, then turned back. "Your Frenchman had best not be at the root of this. And another thing, William. William, look at me."

Beaumont looked up from the instruments he was drying. Pearce gestured at the wounded man.

"You talk to *me* first before you move *him* anywhere. Clear?"

"Yes, Captain. That's clear."

Beaumont slept the remains of that night in a chair beside the wounded man. Sometime between the time when he last checked on the wounded man and sunrise, the man died. A somber group of his fellows from his brigade led in the man's bride, a Fox Indian, a striking beauty, no more that fourteen. Beaumont recognized her from the vaccinations three years past. The girl stood mutely beside the bed, her hands cradling her gravid belly, the outline of her navel visible beneath her thin cotton dress. She leaned in close as if to feel the breath of the man upon her cheek, looked at the voyageurs and Beaumont and Farnham, and then she walked away sobbing.

{ FOURTEEN }

IN THE COLD GRAY DAWN BEAUMONT made his slow, solitary way along the hard-packed path to his cottage. A dusting of snow had fallen. Low flat clouds in the far eastern sky glowed pink. A large bird made its slow flight toward the treetops. From the bushes at the forest edge came the full-throated call of birds, and three smaller birds raced out to harass the large bird. Its long wings beat like oars as it soared upward and away until it was a mere speck above the harbor.

Beaumont had seen the Indian girl before, and she affected him now as when he first met her at the company warehouse. He was in no hurry to return home. He stood along the hilltop facing southeast. Rex was beside him. Someone had wrapped a red kerchief around the dog's neck, and from time to time, he raised one of his hind legs to scratch at it. Beaumont squatted down and untied the kerchief and shook it out into its full dimensions.

He looked down at the dog.

"Everyone takes care of you," he told the dog. "You're lucky."

Other men made great study of the Indians. Crooks speculated often about the origins of the Sioux's blood lust, the independence of the Fox and the sagacity of the Chippewa. For Beaumont the Indians blurred together, the tribes indistinguishable one from the other. The girl, however, he remembered. He had vaccinated her skinny arm some three years ago and saw her each season when the Fox came to collect their tribe's fees. She was beautiful and she was brave, unafraid to scorn with a withering gaze the lecherous soldiers, voyageurs and the company clerks. It saddened him to see her crying as she stood before her beloved, mutilated and rigid in death. The facts of the evening were unknown, but the idea that Alexis was involved sickened him.

When he admitted himself to his house, he found Deborah seated at the kitchen table drinking a cup of milk. Dressed in her nightshirt, cap and stockings, she sat with her back to the low fire, her elbows upon the table-top, her hands about the cup.

"Are you well?" His expression was cast in worry.

"I'm fine." She set down the cup and patted the space on the bench beside her. "Come sit."

"How long have you been up?"

"Since the hour the soldiers came to fetch you. I couldn't fall back asleep."

"Is Sarah up?"

"Asleep."

He eased himself beside her, rubbed his face with his hands, put his arm around her waist and leaned his head upon her shoulder.

"You should get back to bed."

"Later. It's good for me to sit like this. Where's Alexis?"

"Captain Pearce has him in the brig."

"Prison?"

He drew out a deep breath. "There was a stabbing last night. He didn't do it. That I am certain of. He's clever and foolish, but he's not violent."

"What happened to the man who was stabbed?"

"It was a complicated wound."

She set down her cup and took up her husband's hands in hers. "I'm sure I'll hear all about it in the coming days. Emilie Crooks is convinced Alexis was one of the vandals who took down their privy. She's asked me when he has time to work if he's so busy drinking and skylarking. William, he's becoming an embarrassment."

"I heard all about her precious privy. She should pay more attention to her boy George if that's her complaint. That lad's discovered the bottle like an Indian."

The trumpet calling reveille carried in from the fort.

Deborah exhaled. "It just doesn't seem worth it."

"What's not worth it?"

"Worth having him about. Alexis. Our salon's little experiment in reading to him seems to have improved his English but not his morals. Poor Sally must be distraught. She invested so much hope in him."

He did not lift his head from her shoulder as he considered her remark. In time, she spoke again.

"Do you see what I mean?"

Beaumont considered her question. "I've—we've—put a lot into that lad, and he's not well yet. I just don't see." He stopped speaking.

"He's well enough to dance," she said plainly.

"Yes, I heard all about that. And to drink." He swiveled upon the bench to better face her. "And chop wood. And sweep the kitchen. He's well enough to do chores."

"William, by the winter there shall be another child in this house. You shall be a father again. The prospect of a long winter with him here among us and the new baby and Sarah, it worries me. You know Sarah's starting to speak French. She seems to understand him when he chatters at her. And you. I heard you last night when they came for you. There was panic in your voice. You're affected by him too."

He surveyed the crowded kitchen, a space smaller even than the cluttered room his mother kept. His counted out the collection of mismatched mugs along the shelf. There were seven. He traced out the image of an old man's profile in the water stain in the ceiling. "What do you mean affected?"

"I mean only to say that since he moved in here, since you started talking about composing his case for that journal, you've become distracted, distant even. Don't mistake me, William, I want you to succeed. Your success is our success, and you've done so well with him, that he does not fully heal is of small matter. Write up what you have for the *Reporter,* and let's let him leave before the freeze."

She looked about the kitchen, then faced her husband.

"Let me start some breakfast," she said.

He rose.

"No, you sit. I'll bring Sarah to you and take care of breakfast, and then I need to get back to the fort. Captain Pearce wants a meeting about the events of last night. I need to get Alexis back before he has him horse-whipped on the parade ground."

A CORPORAL ADMITTED BEAUMONT into the captain's office. The captain sat behind his desk, cleared of all objects save his short quill, an unlit candle in a pewter stand, an ink bottle and his sword. His cheeks glowed with a fresh shave, and his hair was combed back in a great wave. Ramsay Crooks was thoroughly relaxed with his massive legs extended and crossed at the ankles, his boots at high polish, arms crossed behind his head. The Reverend James sat stiff in his seat.

The captain cleared his throat. "Doctor, I seem to recall a gathering of the same principals assembled here many months ago, and now we're all once again gathered by the river. You well know what happened last night. The voyageurs had their Gumbo ball, words were exchanged, and a man took a knife. And at the center of it all was your Frenchman with the hole in his side.

"Seems that early in the evening his brother Edouard saw fit to make the man a kind of circus show and took bets on how much whiskey Alexis could drink. You know the rest. The lad gulps it down and then slips it out his bunghole. Word got out about his trick, and a couple of St. Louis brigade fellas who lost some cash made a joke of Alexis. Called him the boy with the asshole in his side and fell into mocking him. Edouard made him into an *affair d'honneur.* They got into fisticuffs.

Within an hour a St. Louis man was found in a pool of bloody mud. You saw the results."

Pearce gazed at his desktop, then looked up.

"Frankly, I'm fed up. Your boy with the hole in his side is more trouble than he's worth. I think I speak for the rest of the island when I say that the lad needs to be gone. If he's well enough to chop wood and drink whiskey like a fish, he's well enough to leave. And if I find he was involved in that stabbing, I'll cast him off personally."

Beaumont was nodding slowly. "Captain, with all due respect, embarrassing as his behavior is . . . "

The captain interrupted. "Shameful, I should say."

"Shameful, embarrassing, be that as it may, it strikes me as an uneven exercise of justice to cast away an innocent man. Can anyone properly vouch if Alexis was even there when the fight happened?"

"He's an instigator."

"He's simply trying to recover and make a living, and I've seen fit to provide him the charity to make that possible. What sense is there to cast him away because others abuse him? I fail to see the logic of that ethic."

Pearce exploded. "Damn you, William Beaumont, that man's a drunk and a drain on this island!" He slammed his fist upon the desktop. "You should be ashamed for harboring him. Ashamed! This isn't the first time he's pulled that drinking stunt, and I have good reason to believe he was among the vandals who stove in the Crooks's privy. Reverend?"

The reverend blinked like a bird.

"Alexis is certainly a kind of instigator, but I am neither a lawyer nor a constable. And yet, his drinking and trickery and malfeasance mar the very charity that you and your wife have given him."

Like a praying mantis, the reverend slowly folded his long fingers into a kind of teepee before his face.

Beaumont swallowed hard. "Captain, Reverend, Alexis St. Martin is my patient. He costs the island nothing, and if his drinking is cause for exile, you'd be left with a garrison of schoolboys and girls. He drinks no more than any other soldier and holds it better than half."

Crooks erupted into laughter. "Am I the only one? Am I?" His face had reddened. He wiped his eyes. "Holds it better than half! Good God, I should think he should hold it better. Or rather should not." He gestured as though possessed by some fit and collapsed back upon his chair.

The reverend spoke up. "Doctor, sentiment for the man clouds your judgment. Were he my servant, I would soundly discipline him."

Captain Pearce nodded. "I've heard enough," he snapped. "Doctor, I've ordered Major Thompson to conduct an inquiry into the events of last night. If I find that your boy was even ten feet from that stabbing, he's gone. Gone, do you hear me?"

"Yes, Captain."

"But never mind the hearing. It's your reputation at stake. Not mine. If you had any sense of propriety, you'd see the sense of discharging this drunk—this instigator—from your household and your charity. I've nothing more to say."

{FIFTEEN}

THE FOUR MEN HAD BEEN LOCKED IN THE CELL since before dawn. Alexis was huddled into a corner on a wooden pallet. He sat with his knees pressed up to his chest and was wrapped in a thin blanket so that only the tip of his long nose and chin were visible. His brother Edouard lay on the opposite pallet, his legs crossed, his arms behind his head. Etienne, a fellow voyageur, lay on the floor. His forearm was slung over his eyes, and he was snoring lightly. Edgar stood with his back to them all, his face pressed to the cold grillwork, his hands wrapped around the vertical iron bars. The voyageurs were still outfitted in their clothes from the previous night's dance, pantaloons and red neck kerchiefs. They stank of whiskey and sweat. They had filled their slops bucket to the brim.

Alexis looked over at his brother. "I'm not a show thing."

Edouard turned his head so as to face his younger brother. "What?" he replied dully.

"I said, I'm not a show thing."

Edouard shrugged. He swung his hips so that he could reach deep into the pocket of his trousers. "Here." He tossed Alexis a small cloth purse of coins. It landed with a dull clunk on the cell's packed earth floor. "I had Pierre place a bet on you. So now you're a rich show thing."

Alexis regarded the purse, and then he bent down, looked inside and clutched it close to his chest under the blanket.

"It came to me as an inspiration," Edouard explained. "You know how I am. You still drunk?"

Alexis closed his right eye, then his left, then opened the right again. "No, but I'm still seeing double. You might have told me."

Edouard shrugged. "And then what? Look, we all made something from it. You got plans to work with that hole?" He pointed at his brother. "You could make some good money with that."

They had done their best to refashion the bandages so that the wound was once again compressed and covered.

"When we get out of here, I'm coming with you."

"Not with that." Edouard regarded his brother for some time. "You had a woman with that like that?"

THE TAKER MADE MAD

83

Alexis blushed.

"Never the mind. I was just wondering. Just keep your shirt on if you do."

The brothers sat in silence. Alexis frowned. He took the purse out and hefted its weight.

"You work for the doctor?" Edouard asked.

"I do chores."

"He pays you? They have good money I bet."

Alexis shrugged his shoulders. "I told you. He takes care of me."

"When you gonna be better?"

Alexis shrugged. "The doctor puts things in, takes things out, looks at it, even put some beef in it, but it still won't heal."

"Beef?"

"As some sort of a plug to close up the hole. Didn't work. Something happened to the beef. It just got a hole cut into it. I never seen a man smile the way he did when he saw that. It was like he was happy it didn't work."

Edouard considered the idea, his brow knit into sharp ridges.

"He treats you well?"

"Sometimes when he's poking into it, I feel faint, and everything goes dark like I'm in a cave. He agreed to sew it up, but I won't let him. I'm afraid when he starts cutting he won't stop." He coughed and picked after something in his hair. "He's a strange man. Very serious, you know, like a priest. His wife's sweet in the way the English can be. The child, she's cute. They're to have another."

Alexis stared off into the gloom.

"I want to go." He shivered and clutched the blanket around his skinny shoulders. "Every day he changes the bandages. Sometimes twice a day. It has gotten smaller. Someday it will close. What choice I got? He saved my life."

Edouard gazed at Edgar, who remained with his face pressed to the cold grillwork. He took up his wooden cup and tossed it at Edgar, who did not flinch when the cup bounced off his back and clattered on to the floor. "God, man, why don't you sit your ass down."

Edgar did not move.

"He deaf?" Edouard St. Martin asked Alexis.

Alexis raised his dark eyes slowly. "No. Just leave him be, Edouard."

Edouard dangled a leg off the cot and nudged Etienne with the heel of his boot. "Etienne, what the fuck are you doing sleeping like we were in camp gazing up at the stars? Do any of you care we've been here for what, six hours?" He sat up on the edge of the cot. He called out. "Hello? Hello? Can we get some breakfast? Hey shit carrier, why don't you ask them to get us breakfast?"

Edgar did not move from his place, but he spoke in a monotone. "You talk to me like that one more time, and I will rip off your nuts and stuff them down your skinny Gumbo throat."

Etienne yawned. "Watch out Edouard, he'll do it," he said plainly. "The man's crazier than a badger in heat."

Edouard looked at his fellow prisoners. "They think one of us stabbed Philippe? By God, the man was fucking that Fox chief's daughter practically in broad daylight on the beach." Edouard laughed. He booted Etienne gently once more. "You heard them, no? She's a shrieker." He mimicked the woman's ecstasy, then stopped and looked at the other men. He turned to his brother. He was serious now. "Alexis, listen to me, we got to get out of here. Where's that doctor of yours?"

Alexis shrugged.

Edgar turned away from the grating. "We were together all the night. After the drinking trick, Alexis and I were at the warehouse drinking."

Edouard cocked his head.

"I'll vouch for that," Edgar said.

Edouard nodded slowly. "Yes," he said tentatively.

"And you came along too. Later, we heard shouting. So we went to see what was the matter. That's when we saw those Indians running. Seven of them. And then we found the wounded voyageur. The one who was stabbed."

Alexis was looking at Edgar. Etienne had risen up. The two men looked at Edouard, and Edouard looked at Edgar.

"Well then," Edouard said. "You saw what you saw."

Edgar nodded. He gestured to Alexis. "I'll take that sack of coins you made off the drinking game."

Edouard sneered, then smiled.

"You crazy, crazy white nigger, you." He signaled to Alexis. "Go on brother, pay up. Give him your purse."

SIXTEEN

IN THE DAYS FOLLOWING THE MEETING in Captain Pearce's office, Beaumont was in a back-and-forth debate with himself about what to do with Alexis. Sometimes, he was determined to send him away. Others, he chided himself for his cowardice and lack of resolve. He opened his notebook to a clean page and drew a large capital *T;* on the one side of it he wrote, "*Al. stays*" and on the other "*Al. leaves.*" Under each heading, he wrote the reasons to support it, but he soon found the exercise futile. The same reasons fit on both sides of his balance sheet: reputation, promotion, Alexis's well-being. It seemed an offense to balance some reasons against others: Deborah's contentment versus income. Perhaps he should pray for guidance, but he had not done such a thing since he was a boy. He looked over Franklin's guide for moral perfection: useless. Perhaps Alexis would be found guilty, and he would have no choice but to send him off. Some days, he regretted he had taken the wounded man from the company store.

A week later, Major Hardage Thompson called Beaumont to his office. He had concluded his investigation.

"I wanted to be the first to tell you this, William. I know how much the lad means to you, so I thought it best I speak to you rather than let rumor or Captain Pearce deliver the news."

The blood was pounding in Beaumont's chest.

The major took up his paper and slipped on his spectacles. He summarized the findings. Edouard St. Martin had indeed offered a bet that his brother could drink more than any other man. But no evidence supported Alexis's involvement in the stabbing. Edgar's testimony was key. He vouched that in the hours before and after the stabbing he and Alexis had been together drinking outside the warehouse. By the hour of the stabbing, they were too drunk to stand. Alexis was exonerated of all involvement in the stabbing.

"Perhaps they fixed their stories, but others corroborate it," Thompson concluded. He removed his spectacles. "Honestly, William, I tried every which way to catch Edgar up, Edouard and Alexis as well, but they were consistent to every detail, even to the number of Indians. Seven, they insist. You know how these men are. Everyone speaks, but no one says anything. It's over. Alexis is a free man. You can take him home now. If you wish."

Beaumont sat expressionless.

"What's wrong, William?"

"I'm like Adam cast from Eden, so ashamed of what I've done."

Thompson lowered his eyes.

"You think so too, don't you?" Beaumont insisted.

The major coughed and smoothed his hands over his thighs. "That you feel simply means you're a man. I know you have a particular attachment to him, that he's become like a son to you. It's hard to see your child go astray, and yet his behavior this summer has been at times, to speak plainly, deplorable. I won't lie to you, friend. Others question the logic of your charity."

"Logic of charity," Beaumont pronounced. "Does such a sentiment have logic? In the war, we would have so many patients, but from time to time, one or another captured our attention more than others. Something in their manner, their illness, the circumstances of their wound, made you pay extra attention. It's like that with Alexis."

Thompson nodded slowly.

"Debbie finds the man crude. Perhaps I should just let him go, but I've invested so much in that lad. As has Sally. What should I do?"

"Honestly, William, you've done your very best for him, and for that you should be proud. You truly have done your best, but now he's become a drain not only upon your charity but I fear also your reputation. Remember the malingering Lieutenant Griswold? Take away a man's reputation, and all that remains is positively bestial. Charity is a limited obligation. You mustn't let it overmaster you."

Beaumont chuckled. "What do you think Ramsay Crooks would do?"

"Ramsay? I expect he'd figure out a way to make some cash off that drinking trick Alexis does."

THAT AFTERNOON BEAUMONT went to the brig to collect Alexis. Two soldiers, each armed with shouldered rifles, led the way. One carried the key ring with great ceremony. Beaumont waited at the edge of the parade ground for the soldiers to return with the freed prisoners.

The three voyageurs walked out in a single file, shivering. Edgar followed behind, costumed in wrappings of furs and blankets sewed up about his thighs and shoulders so that he looked like a scarecrow outfitted for the freeze. His feet and legs were slipped into crude stockings fashioned from the length of some animal's leg fur turned inside out and cinched at the ends of his feet, creating the effect of a jester's fur-lined booties. Edgar hopped from one foot to the other, looked at Edouard, then turned and trotted across the parade grounds to the gates to the fort.

The three voyageurs just stood there. Etienne scratched at his head, drew something out between his fingertips and inspected his discovery.

Alexis gazed at his oversized shoes. Edouard, looking after Edgar, chuckled and announced that the man was a lunatic. Beaumont stood before them, his hands in his coat pockets.

Alexis gestured shyly to his brother.

"Doctor, this is my brother Edouard."

Beaumont extended his right hand.

"Edouard. Good to meet you."

Edouard stepped forward, clasped Beaumont's hand between his and pumped it vigorously. "Dr. Beaumont. Alexis has told me all about you. You, sir, you are his savior. On behalf of the entire St. Martin family, we salute you, Doctor, and say that we are forever your humble servants." He affected a small bow. "What you have done is nothing short of a miracle. A miracle. If ever we can repay you, you have only to ask."

Beaumont drew his hand away. "Thank you," he said.

Edouard continued. "Let me present our comrade Etienne Desauliers of Montreal, a fellow Blackfeather like Alexis and myself."

Etienne nodded civilly as he shook Beaumont's hand.

"Well, gentlemen, you're all free men again," Beaumont announced. "It's late, Alexis, and it's been a long week for us. Let's go home. Deborah and Sarah are worried about you. We'll change your dressings and get you in some warm clothes." He made a gesture for Alexis to follow him.

Alexis did not move. He looked to Edouard, then to Etienne, but both men stood poker faced. Alexis started to speak to them in French.

Edouard cut him off. "Go on little brother, do as your doctor says. Your bandages need changing. But here, first."

Edouard held open his arms and embraced Alexis. He told Alexis he loved him and would see him in the spring. Etienne did the same. The four men crossed the parade ground to the gate together, and then the two voyageurs walked downhill to their crowded camp on the beach, and Alexis and Beaumont returned to their small house at the edge of the village. Halfway there, Beaumont draped his right arm over Alexis's shoulders and drew him close.

SEVENTEEN

FOR WEEKS, BEAUMONT IGNORED ALEXIS. He put away his notebook, shelved Brown's *Elementa Medicinae* and ceased gazing into the wound and collecting gastric liquor with his gum elastic tube. The mere sight of the Frenchman was enough to incite him to a simmering, square-jawed anger.

Some days, Beaumont wanted Alexis to leave. He wanted to beg Deborah's forgiveness for his selfishness and neglect of his duties to her and their family. He wanted to tell Captain Pearce that his sentiment of mercy for this wounded Gumbo had overcome his right reason. Other days, he imagined himself in Paris, at the center of an operating theater, demonstrating Alexis's wound, displaying the process of digestion, holding up a vial of the clear gastric liquor, explaining the action of the stomach to an assembly of physicians. This longing and the impossibility of ever achieving it, they drew him to despair.

One afternoon, as he sat in his darkening office staring out the window, he decided Alexis must go. Deborah would be happy, he would write the case report as best he could, his reputation would be repaired.

As he was convincing himself this was the proper course of action, a knock came at his door.

"Enter," he called.

Captain Pearce and Brevet Major Hardage Thompson stepped into the room.

"Pardon the disturbance, Doctor," the captain announced. "I see you enjoying the darkness here. Interesting. But I bring a certain sort of light. News from Washington City." He produced a packet of papers from his coat pocket and set them on the tabletop.

Thompson sat. The captain looked over at him but said nothing. He took up the paper.

"It's an order from Washington City. From President Monroe. Allow me, please." The captain paused to scan the page. Thompson was staring blankly into the space of Beaumont's cluttered desk.

"*I, President James Monroe, Commander in Chief of the U.S. Army, restore Lieutenant Edmond B. Griswold to his rank of Second Lieutenant with all pay and privileges as appropriate to that rank and owed from the date of his arrest.*"

Beaumont was wide-eyed. "What in God's name?"

"There's more, Doctor." The captain looked at Thompson, then continued to read. *"The evidence before the court did not warrant the decision it rendered. The conviction rests on testimony from one Assistant Surgeon William Beaumont whose evidence is more an expression of his professional opinion than a statement of facts. Moreover, this opinion is shaken by the testimony from fellow officers Lieutenants Russell and Morris who stated that Lieutenant Griswold could not perform his duties because he was ill. The testimony of Brevet-Major Thompson and that of Assistant Surgeon Beaumont both bear internal marks of excited feelings, impairing their credibility.*

"Assistant Surgeon Beaumont is to be especially singled out for making an experiment upon his patient of more than doubtful propriety in the relations of a medical advisor to his patient. A medicine of violent operation, administered by a physician to a man whom he believes to be in full health, but who is taking his professional advice, is a very improper test of the sincerity of the patient's complaints, and the avowal of it as a transaction justifiable in itself discloses a mind warped by ill will, or insensitive to its own relative duties."

The captain held the paper before him by his thumb and forefinger. "It's signed President James Monroe and dated the 3rd of September 1823," he said flatly as he let it drop like a dry leaf on to the tabletop.

Pearce's manner became unusually sympathetic. "I'll leave this with you to review. Good day." The scrape and step of his boots came heavy upon the floorboards.

THOMPSON WAS DEVASTATED. "What're we going to do?"

Beaumont held the paper like some condemned man reviewing his warrant. His hands shook and then too his jaw. He said slowly, "If I had this case to do again and to do again a hundred times, I would do exactly as I have done." He looked at Thompson. "We shall defend our honor."

"How?" Thompson had covered his face with his hands. "Challenge James Monroe to pistols at thirty paces?"

"A court of inquiry into the matter. I shall demand a court of inquiry be formed and the matter reviewed by my peers. Medical peers. Hardage, look at me. Please."

Thompson lowered his hands.

"This is my problem, not yours. I must take the weight of this. I'll speak with Captain Pearce straightaway to initiate the court."

"I think he wishes the thing be done and gone."

"The thing has just begun, Hardage."

Thompson wiped his eyes with the back of his hand. "I can't bear to walk about the garrison with this cloud over my name. I feel positively bestial." He began sobbing.

"Hardage, compose yourself. I share your disgust but not your shame. My reputation is dear to me too."

Thompson's face was tear stained. "If only you hadn't given the man that dose."

Beaumont slapped the tabletop. "And if only you had forced lieutenants Russell and Morris, your two fancy academy men, to submit their testimony, we'd not be sitting here like some pair of fools sharing a presidential rebuke."

"William Beaumont, are ambition and anger the only emotions you feel?"

Beaumont's ears reddened. "Hardage, what the devil?"

"You could have . . ."

Beaumont interrupted him. "Could have what?" he yelled. "What precisely? *What?* You came to me distressed about the man, and I did my duty. Now you sit here and sob like a woman in a calico dress. Wipe your nose, and act like a man."

"For God's sake, William, the man's father's a judge out east."

Beaumont snapped. "That has nothing to do with it!"

Thompson exploded. "Why is everything always such a matter of high-minded principle with you? Why? You said to me you felt doubt. That very day. You said you felt doubt about your so-called diagnosis."

Beaumont took in a great breath. He gazed at the ceiling, then looked at Hardage and spoke evenly. "Doubt? Then that's my third emotion. No, fourth. Disgust too. The truth shall win out and restore our reputations. This is a medical matter. Why the president of the United States chooses to involve himself I cannot fathom. I've copied out some fourteen pages in my notebook of cases of malingering. With all due respect to our commander in chief, just as I presume not to manage his practice as president, he cannot mine as physician."

Beaumont paused.

"Hardage, look at me. Look at me, please. The only thing we can do is show some pluck and fight this, not each other. Do you have some other idea?"

The major shook his head slowly, then rose and walked out of the office. Beaumont called after him, following him to the threshold of the hospital. He would have chased him down, but the sight of passersby watching caused him to retreat to his office. He closed the door and sat heavily in his chair. As he gazed upon the president's order, he considered the tiny initials of the clerk who had dutifully copied these devastating words: this document was one of many in that clerk's work committing other men's words to paper, a humble job, without tribulation, but with a steady income.

LATE IN THE AFTERNOON, Beaumont called on Captain Pearce. The captain was at his desk, wiping the octagonal barrel of his gun with a soft oiled cloth. His uniform coat was slung over the back of his chair, and his shirt-sleeves were rolled up above his elbows. A glass of whiskey sat before him. He glanced at Beaumont, then returned to his gun.

"I'm sorry about the order," he said. "Reasonable people will disagree."

"Captain, my reputation is dear to me. It is truly all that I have. I should like to petition to the adjutant general for a court of inquiry into the matter."

The captain shrugged. He took up a rigid brass cleaning rod, wrapped a small square of green felt about the tip, then began to carefully pass the felt through the length of the barrel. "Go on then."

"A court of inquiry composed of medical men and candid judges who are equipped to properly review the facts of the matter and decide whether what was done was mere opinion or, as I submit, a statement of medical fact legitimately gathered."

"I'll not stop you from writing for such a hearing."

"But will you support it, Captain?"

The captain set the gun down, then looked directly at Beaumont. "No."

Beaumont did not remove his gaze from the captain, nor did the captain remove his from Beaumont.

"Why, sir?"

"Because the commander in chief has spoken, and I'll not protest against his orders."

"Captain, this is not a protest. It's a petition and . . ."

The captain cut him off. "Don't get Jesuitical with me, Assistant Surgeon William Beaumont! I can call on His Holiness Father Didier if I so desire that. I'm a soldier charged with policing this garrison so that peace reigns and thus commerce thrives. That's peacetime in a democracy for you."

The captain curled his lip. "This is your private affair. Just like your devotion to that drunken Gumbo with the hole in his side." He shook his head slowly. "Like a dog to his vomit, so a fool returns to his folly. There's something to be learned from this, I'd reckon, but I'm not a clergyman. I thought you all had some sort of ethic about doing no harm, but you, sir, have a queer sort of ethic, near poisoning a soldier, then exhausting your charity and reputation on some useless fur trapper with a bunghole in his side. But I'll leave such inquiries with the likes of our good Reverend James, or Father Didier when he comes to wet the brown babies' heads, but there is something to be learned." The captain chuckled. "Good day to you, Doctor." He gestured with the gun to the door to his office.

THAT EVENING, AFTER ALEXIS had gone out, while Sarah slept in her cradle, Beaumont and Deborah sat together at the kitchen table. She set down her sewing. "What's wrong? You've been quiet all evening."

He sighed. "Have you heard the latest news of the Griswold matter?"

She shook her head.

When he finished the story, she stammered, then rose to hug her husband. "William, this is terrible. Terrible."

He tried to soothe her.

"I debated even telling you, but it's better that you hear this from me than from the gossips of the island. I know how word gets about."

"The president of the United States," she said.

"Deborah, please don't upset yourself. It's all a misunderstanding. Clearly lieutenants Russell and Morris made a case out of this. Now I understand why they insisted on being transferred to Detroit. I was neither advised nor consulted about the appeal. Had the president consulted me or any other like-minded medical man, he'd have understood that this is a medical matter and that I comported myself with the utmost professional judgment. Deborah, please, my love, don't weep."

"It's so awful. What did he say? A mind warped, not sensitive to your duties? What will this do to your prospects for promotion to surgeon?"

"Warped by ill will. It's just rhetoric to make a case, but plainly it's not a case well made. Now please, sit. You mustn't strain yourself."

He eased her to her seat.

"Your promotion?"

He stroked her hair. "I will solve this. It's all my doing. My mistake. I should have simply let the man wallow in his melancholy. I was too much possessed to do what was right, too disturbed at how he was using me to excuse his sloth, too moved by Hardage's appeal to me for help. And now it has cost me my friendship with Hardage. That I do regret."

"Why not just say that then?"

"Say what?"

"To Hardage, to the president. Say that you were too much possessed by your high moral principles. Not to argue, but to ask for their mercy."

He stared at her. "I can't do that now, Debbie. I can't. I must fight back, to maintain my reputation. I've already begun composing a letter petitioning for a court of inquiry into the matter, composed of my peers and fair judges. In time, this'll all be rectified and my name cleared. All of this will be forgotten as so many misunderstandings are forgotten. Time's a queer thing, Deborah. There's the truth, and then there's the memory of the truth."

He held her closer.

"You know, that play we read this summer. The *Midsummer Night's*

Dream, the one with people transformed into animals. I think about the play and us on this island and wonder if we're not being taunted by fairies spinning fortune's wheel and playing with our dreams, showing us for the fools we are."

"And Alexis is Puck?" She smiled. "Here to make us mad."

"But we're not fools, Deborah."

"We think we can control what we want, work for it, but fate overrules us and drives us mad. After Nathaniel betrayed me and I returned in shame to my father's house, I learned that the best we can do is to steady ourselves, live simply and hope for God's mercy."

"And then I appeared."

"That is my point. My mercy and trust were rewarded."

"Don't worry, Deborah. In time, we'll be gone from this place, living in a fine home, in a civilized town. I know what I must do: finish the case report and submit it to Surgeon General Lovell. I'll ask his guidance on publishing it. With a case worthy of the *Medical Recorder,* I'll surely have his support, as well as the support of the surgeon general's corps. When Lovell sees that case, I'm certain he will support my promotion. That case shall more than counterbalance whatever stain the Griswold affair leaves upon my reputation."

He did not work on the case report and the letter to Lovell. Instead, he wrote and rewrote his petition for an appeal of the president's judgment upon his professional character. He saved the drafts in chronological order. The document ran to five neatly scripted pages. After he posted it in the mail pack to Detroit, he rose each and every morning anticipating a reply. When that reply finally came, it was only a single sentence.

"The petition by Assistant Surgeon William Beaumont on behalf of Assistant Surgeon William Beaumont has neither standing nor merit and is thus denied."

BEAUMONT GREW DESPONDENT.

Deborah was soon to deliver. Alexis returned later and later in the evenings, always intoxicated. Hardage Thompson would no longer speak with him, his wife, Sally, avoided him, and the Reverend James, his wife, and Emilie Crooks treated him with cold civility. Captain Pearce regarded him with mocking disdain. Deborah's pregnancy soon became a convenient excuse for them to decline invitations to dinner, to leave a sociable early. Only Ramsay Crooks seemed unchanged. He found the whole set of events amusing.

"The ladies' reading experiment seems to have been a bit of a bust," he announced one afternoon when he encountered Beaumont as Beaumont was leaving the company store with a boxful of supplies.

The nightmares of Beaumont's youth returned. The barn door was left open, and the cows were lost. His father was in a simmering square-jawed rage. Some nights he didn't sleep, and on those when he did, he often awoke in confusion and terror; the pale light of the bedroom window was not where it should be, and the dresser beside the bed he shared with his brothers had vanished, and then he recovered his wits and calmed himself that he was not in Lebanon, Connecticut, with his brothers beside him snoring and dreaming, but beside his wife in their modest house on Mackinac Island.

Twice, Beaumont nearly ordered Alexis out of the house, but both times he changed his mind. He looked again at the table he had made of reasons for and against Alexis's departure. He took up his pencil and scribbled out the words "*Alexis leaves*" in great jagged, sweeping strokes, like the kind his daughter Sarah made at play with a carbon pencil, then circled "*Alexis stays.*"

He was not only convinced it was essential to keep Alexis, but he had also begun to believe it was better that the wound remained open. He tried to banish this thought as soon as it arose, but it came again, like lust, and each time it returned it was more demanding and powerful and undeniable. He could not banish what he had learned over the last year: Alexis was a living laboratory, and he was his. As he considered the observations and experiments he might perform on him, he was suspended between the poles of enthusiasm and despair. He had not the slightest experience or skill to perform experiments. The more he observed Alexis's stomach, the less he understood.

He decided he needed Surgeon General Lovell's support to continue with his experiments. That support would not only cover the stain of the Griswold affair, but also give him time to conduct the experiments while he still earned his forty dollars a month income as an assistant surgeon.

November 1823.
Dear Doctor Lovell,
    I write to you with news of a most interesting case for your consideration. Since, June of 1822, I have cared for a lad, a fur trapper, who was accidentally shot by the unlucky discharge of a gun. The whole charge, consisting of powder and duck shot, was received in the left side at no more than 2 or 3 feet distance from the muzzle of the piece, carrying away by its force the integuments more than the size of the palm of a man's hand. Accompanying this letter is a thorough summary of my successful efforts with the case that I humbly suggest may be worthy for publication in the Medical Reporter.
    Within nine months, the lad had recovered perfect health and a hardy,

robust constitution, able to perform any kind of labor from the whittling of a stick to the chopping of logs, but the wound still remains with an aperture to the man's stomach. When he lies on the opposite side I can look directly into the cavity, and almost see the process of digestion. I can pour in water with a funnel, or put food in with a spoon, and draw them out again with a siphon. I have frequently suspended flesh, raw and wasted, and other substances, into the perforation to ascertain the length of time required to digest each; and at one time used a tent of raw beef, instead of lint, to stop the orifice, and found that in less than five hours it was completely digested off, as smooth and even as if it had been cut with a knife.

The case affords an excellent opportunity for experimenting upon the gastric fluids and process of digestion. It would give no pain, nor cause the least uneasiness, to extract a gill of fluid every two or three days, for it frequently flows out spontaneously in considerable quantities. Various kinds of digestible substances might be introduced into the stomach, and then easily examined during the whole process of digestion. I may therefore be able hereafter to give some interesting experiments on these subjects.

> *Sincerely,*
> *Wm. Beaumont*
> *Assistant Surgeon, US Army*

❦{EIGHTEEN}❧

BY THE END OF NOVEMBER, the population of the beach had dwindled to just a few tents and lean-tos as the voyageurs and Indians broke camp and packed their possessions into bateaux and canoe. They rose at daybreak and gathered at the shoreline to survey the horizon, the clouds and wind to judge whether to depart for the mainland. Small waves chattered at their feet.

Deborah was confined to bed. Her legs had swollen so that Beaumont could pit his thumb into the soft white flesh about her ankles as if it were dough. Mrs. Farnham had charge of Sarah. When she and the child left the house on errands, Alexis remained in case Deborah began her labor. Beaumont kept at his work. He had to. The sick rolls were steady with an intermittent fever, and Emilie Crooks had a new set of pains. One week, he called on her almost daily.

In mid-December, the first of the winter storms came around noon. It began as flakes floating like soft feathers and settling upon men's caps and shoulders, then increased to a steady snow that became sheets of pelting needles that pricked the raw skin of a man's cheek. The snow continued for hours, overnight and through the second day. On the third day, when Alexis tried the door to the house, it gave way only a few inches before it met a dead weight like pushing against sacks of grain.

The storm and the winds that followed the storm kept them winter-locked for days. Deborah read Rousseau's *Julie,* a gift from Emilie Crooks. In the evening, William read aloud the poems of Burns. Sarah traced her small fingers over the woodcut prints that illustrated the poems and asked her father for stories about the lambs and the farmers and the fish. Alexis kept to his small room or squatted upon a stool before the kitchen fire, smoking a short clay pipe and whittling as he listened to the stories. Beaumont cooked a venison stew that lasted them for three days. Some nights were so cold that the bowls of their spoons steamed like living beings.

ONE EVENING, AFTER SUPPER, as Beaumont was dressing Alexis's wound, Deborah called to him from the bedroom. "William, can you come?"

He looked at Alexis, hesitating.

"William, I need *you,*" she yelled.

THE TAKER MADE MAD

97

In haste, he rose up, telling Alexis to just lie there. He found Deborah in their bedroom, squatting, breathing fast, panting, her dress and the floor about soaked as if she had pissed herself.

"Deborah," he cried.

She moaned. "This is the only position." She pressed her head against her crossed arms upon the wall and resumed panting.

He stood behind her with his hands on her shoulders. "Alexis," he shouted.

"William," she moaned. "It hurts like a fire in my bowels will explode. Get Helen Farnham."

"Let's get you in to bed."

"Now, William. Now!"

He shouted again for Alexis. The lad did not appear.

"Where in God's name are you, boy?"

He turned, and there was Alexis at the doorway, shirtless as Beaumont had left him. The violaceous pucker of his wound was visible like some errantly placed anus. His expression that of a spooked deer.

"Fetch Mrs. Farnham. Double time. Use my snowshoes if you require them. Go. Go quickly!"

Three hours later, Deborah delivered her second child. A boy they named William.

The next evening, the two men sat alone at the kitchen table eating dinner. The low fire and the lantern cast their faces in shadows.

"Will she live?" Alexis asked.

Beaumont slowed his chewing as he studied his plate.

"My mother, she died after she delivered my third sister, Emiline. I was just a boy. It was the winter like now. Blood and everything. It was horrible." Alexis's voice trailed off.

Beaumont set down his utensils. He reached for the pitcher of water and began filling his glass. "They always bleed. They need to. It's Nature's manner of restoring the body to its equilibrium. Mrs. Beaumont will live."

"Good." Alexis drummed the tabletop with his fingers. "You know, Doctor, when you called me I was not able to come right away because I was without my dressings and I'd eaten. I feared that if I stood, food would spill out. But when you called again, I got up and I came. I heard how much you needed me."

"You don't have to apologize, Alexis. It was frightening."

"Thank you, Doctor. Nothing at all was left. All of the sudden it was all gone like that." He snapped his fingers.

Beaumont regarded Alexis. "Nothing came out? Out of the hole?"

Alexis nodded, and then he shrugged his shoulders. "Nothing at all. It was all gone. Incredible."

"Did it hurt?"

"Only when you put in that tube to drain the fluid does it hurt."

"No, when you got up. Did your stomach hurt? The wound?"

Alexis shook his head.

Beaumont stood up and took up the lamp.

"Let's go to your room and have a look."

Beaumont gestured to the door. The lamplight cast his shadow large and shimmering behind him.

Alexis lay back, and Beaumont cut away the dressing and lifted off the compress. The hole was as it always was. In the last few weeks, a small fold or doubling of the gastric coats, the size of a silver dollar, pink and moist as a dog's tongue, had appeared and begun to cover the hole. It yielded to gentle digital pressure and did not at all intrude on Beaumont's inspection of the gastric contents. There it was again. Beaumont pressed the forefinger of his right hand against this tissue, and it gave way to expose the cavity and the scent of the evening's meal. He withdrew the finger, and the fold of tissue reappeared. Beaumont asked Alexis to sit up.

"Now?"

"Yes, up here now, on the edge of the bed. Here." Beaumont patted the edge of the bed.

Alexis slowly eased himself upward, and as he did a spurt of brown liquid shot out from the hole like ejaculate. Alexis cursed, but Beaumont put his hand squarely against the small of his back to keep him from lying back on the bed in the customary posture for inspection of his wound. Alexis whimpered like a child and cupped his hands over the hole as if to catch the egress of his meal. He held his hands before the wound, and then he slowly raised them outward and upward in a vague gesture as if to fly.

The hole was sealed.

"Stay like that," Beaumont commanded.

He reached for the lamp and leaned in closely to inspect the hole. The space was filled by a protrusion of pink flesh now acting as a kind of valve. He pushed his finger into that flesh. It was tense, surely holding in the contents of the evening's meal.

Beaumont studied the wound. "Lie back," he commanded.

Alexis did as he was ordered.

Beaumont pushed with his finger and the pink flap gave way again. His forefinger freely entered the cavity as far as his second knuckle. The inside felt warm and wet with the evening meal. He drew his finger out and wiped it with a cloth.

"Now up again. Up."

This time Alexis rose slowly. The fold of gastric tissue had settled into place and covered the hole, a kind of natural lid.

Alexis stood, all the while gazing at the wound. His long greasy black hair hung about his face. He cupped his hands before it in anticipation of an efflux of gastric contents. Nothing came. He looked at his hands, looked at Beaumont, who gazed at the orifice that was no longer a simple orifice.

"*Oh, mon dieu.*" Alexis crossed himself. "I'm cured. Dr. Beaumont, I am cured. You are my savior." He began to weep.

NINETEEN

FOR WEEKS FOLLOWING HER DELIVERY, Deborah kept to bed. When she tried to walk, the throbbing pains in her swollen legs were so great that she moaned and shuffled back to bed. Beaumont wished to bleed her, but she demurred and only allowed him to wrap her calves with elastic dressings. She took her meals in bed, cradled the infant William and nursed him. Sarah lay beside her, gazing at her nursing infant brother.

In the evenings, Beaumont listened to her stories of her childhood when she lived at her father's hotel and she and her sisters helped to care for their infant siblings. He listened as her voice thickened and slowed until sleep overcame her. He lay awake or sat in the chair as he rocked the infant, stroking his tiny back as he analyzed the development of the orifice's valvular flap.

The event reminded him of patients who presented to his surgery with an ulcer the size of a half eagle dollar, an appendage swollen to twice its natural dimensions, or skin the color of a new race of men. When he asked these patients as plain and matter-of-fact as he could, *when did this start,* they hesitated, shrugged, they couldn't honestly say how long; just the other day they had noticed it.

So it had been with the flap of gastric lining over the hole in Alexis's wound. When did it start? Perhaps it had slowly developed over the past weeks. The tissues of the wound were like the pattern of sand, stones and jetsam along the lakeshore, ever changing and, after the storm of an infection or a debridement, entirely rearranged. Now, there it was. A lid over the hole.

That chance, rather than his careful observation, had revealed the flap's significance bothered Beaumont. This wound was not only Alexis's wound, but his as well. His side had the same puckered orifice, the same cicatricle swirl of scar tissue that he had come to accept as simply a natural part of him. This fold of tissue the size of his thumbnail changed everything. The tissues still needed to be observed, the flap could change, but the need to dress the wound daily with a tight compress was gone. Alexis was, in a manner of speaking, cured.

BY THE END OF JANUARY, the thin skin of Deborah's eyelids had wrinkled and darkened to the color of buff kid leather, the hair about her temples had thinned, and dry gray strands were visible amid her auburn hair. The bones of her feet were once again visible, and she could wear her shoes without pain.

At Fort Hill, weeks living in close quarters and days so cold the piss in the tin pots outside the laundry froze solid began to affect the soldiers' health. The count of men on the sick roll grew. Men came on, came off it, and some returned sicker than when the fever had first struck them. Some of the men developed a high fever with soaking sweats and rattling in the chest, with phlegm the color of rust. These Beaumont treated with the lancet and blistering clysters over the congested region.

One evening, Beaumont returned early from the hospital. Deborah was cooking a joint of beef over a low kitchen fire, the fat dripping and flaming. Sarah was stacking wooden blocks on the hearth. Alexis was out. Beaumont sat with his legs stretched out so that his stocking feet warmed, his boots upright beside them.

Deborah sat beside her husband. "You look tired."

He gazed into the fire. "Well as common. Where's Alexis?"

"I let him go after his afternoon chores. Did you see him at the fort?"

"Saw him about the company warehouses earlier today, tossing snowballs with some of the clerks. How's he here with you?"

She shrugged. "Fine. He does his chores, and then he's off and back more or less when he promises. Red nosed sometimes, but he's back. I suppose he prepares us for life with a son."

Beaumont shook his head slowly. "Not that lad. You don't read to him anymore, do you?"

She shook her head. "Not since the time of my confinement. With Sarah wanting attention and walking it was hard."

"I remember when Sally Thompson and you read to him in the hospital from the children's primer. Does he read? That Bible he keeps? Crooks's gift, if you can fathom that."

She shook her head. "He's not literate. I think he just keeps it, like a kind of treasure. Our experiment in moral improvement seems a failure."

"That's what Ramsay says."

The two of them gazed at the cooking beef.

"How is he?" she asked. "You're not so intent on checking the wound twice a day."

Beaumont took up one of his boots, inspected an imperfection in its stitching and then began to slip it on. "He's doing well. The wound's formed a sort of flap over the hole. It's a tiny bit of tissue, and that works well to seal the thing closed. Well enough that he no longer needs the compress dressing."

She set down her fork. "You mean he's healed?"

"In a manner of speaking, I suppose, yes."

"William, that's wonderful. You must be so proud."

"Proud?"

"You healed him. It's been what, nearly two years, and now he's as he was before the injury."

"Not at all as he was. That hole still remains."

"That explains so why he's so changed in his countenance and manner. He's like a boy again. Sometimes, I hear him singing hymns."

Beaumont took a pewter cup from a peg, stepped over to a short barrel of cider and poured out a cup to warm beside the fire. "It's simply a clever fold of gastric tissue that Nature managed upon its own."

Deborah stepped closer to her husband. "But you did it. Nature takes nurture, and you provided that. What will happen to him now?"

"What will happen?"

"He's healed, has he not?"

"It's only a valve, not a seal. Though I don't need to bind the wound closed with that complicated dressing, with minimal effort I can still gain access into the cavity. He can get up and walk about and do his chores."

Deborah was confused. "But why would he?"

"Why would he get up?"

"Why would he stay here? He's a fur trapper. I'd expect he'd want to be rid of this place the moment the ice clears."

"Has he spoken of this to you?"

"The wound?"

"No. Leaving in the spring."

"Of course not, William. William, what's the matter? What's wrong?"

"He may no longer need the compress and in a sense is healed, but let's not go calling a man with a persistent fistula into his stomach cured simply because he does not need a compress dressing to close it."

"William, you needn't raise your voice."

"I'm not raising my voice."

"You are."

He closed his eyes. How to be Resolute and yet Tranquil? When he spoke it was near a whisper. "His fistula remains, and I can't predict what shape it may take in the coming months. As long as I can gain access into his stomach, I have every intention of continuing my study. He may wish to leave, but he mustn't. I need him. We need him. By Heaven, I was the one who nursed him from the brink of death, who changed his dressing twice a day, who took him in and assumed all costs of his care when the leaders of this town saw fit to cast him away in a boat. I know precisely the fate of such men. I saw it in the war."

Deborah regarded her husband, and he her. He reached for his mug but then drew back. His hand was trembling. "Forgive me for raising my voice."

She swallowed hard. "Of course. Of course I do."

"You must know that Alexis is more than a singular case. Much more. The entire process of human digestion is here before me to be observed, studied and experimented upon. This is a once-in-a-lifetime opportunity. Sometimes I think to myself that it's like the land out west. If I don't claim it, someone else surely will. Should I just let him go, the first doctor who has a bit of common sense will see what opportunity lies in the study of him.

"Here on this island is the greatest opportunity to study the process of human digestion. I can't just let him leave and end up with another physician. I've told you before, most surely I'll hear that physician's laughter clear across the country at the folly of the man who sent this prize off in a bateau."

"William, what is it that you propose?"

"I don't know, Deborah. I do know there is an opportunity here that I cannot ignore. I need time to think about what to do. How to do it. When he lies on his side I can look directly into the cavity and almost see the process of digestion. I've suspended flesh into it, raw meat, and seen it dissolve. It takes near thirty minutes for raw beef. Deborah, I've seen things no other physician has seen. I've seen wonderful things. Don't you see?"

"You're a physician, William."

"I know what I am."

"You're physician to the garrison and borough of Mackinac. You're continually pressed with work. How then can you propose to study this man and his stomach?"

"There will be time, there will be time. I beg you, Deborah, just to give me time. I've sent a letter to Dr. Lovell presenting the case and the proposal to perform experiments."

"What did you propose?"

"Deborah, when it is done . . . "

"When what is done? What?"

"When my study of digestion is done, I shall have knowledge that will change the field of medicine. You see how the men eat and drink with intemperate dissipation unto dissolution, farced with crude food, coming about with moans and groans and all kinds of pains and lamentations. I will have the knowledge about how we digest what we eat. Not only the army will value such knowledge, but all people will. Everyone eats.

"The results will be splendid. A book to sell thousands of copies. Here and in Europe. Akin to Franklin's *Experiments and Observations on Electricity*, but grander. Far grander. With that kind of recognition, the Griswold affair will be forgotten. I'd have my pick of posts. We could well be in St. Louis, or even Plattsburgh, well settled, and comfortable in our means. All I ask, Deborah, is your patience to keep the man here. I know it's a burden on you. On us. He's odd, to be sure, but it's a burden we share as we share its reward.

"But what if he won't agree to this plan?"

"I can't imagine Lovell would disagree."

"No, I meant Alexis. What if he won't agree?"

"Why would he not? I've cared for him for more than a year and a half now. He owes his life to me. All I'm asking of him is a small measure of gratitude. He trusts me, and he needs me."

He hesitated.

"Alexis is my hope. Our hope. Especially now, after the president's rebuke. I tell you, in time, his case shall be known the world over. What's happening now reminds me of my years as an apprentice to Chandler. And my years in the war. Some days were like years. At the end of a week, I'd look at my notebook and wonder who I was at the beginning of the week. That's how much I had learned. Do you believe me, do you trust me, Deborah?"

She studied her husband. This manner of conversation, her honest plea and his answer, it had occurred only once before, and that man had betrayed her. Now, sitting in the kitchen of her small house, she realized that the moment to change things had already passed. She told her husband she trusted him. She had no choice. She was bound to his choice.

They embraced.

"Trust me, Debbie. My father left me only debts. I intend to leave my family wealth. Someday we shall have a grand house of our own. Someday we shall have all the things we desire. Like the Crookses."

{TWENTY}

WINTER EXHAUSTED HIM. Both its labors and its loneliness. Some days he dreamed of the book about digestion; others, he dreaded the project. He kept to his notebooks, jotting notes and ideas, rereading past entries. *"Tended to a young voyageur at the company's store. Shot into his left lower chest. Accident. Wound engages both lung & stomach, likely mortal."* He understood why some men drank to forget.

By April, the ice began to melt enough that it was no longer safe to ice fish and, after a week so warm that men were in shirtsleeves by noon, boats began to appear in the harbor, at first singly, but soon in groups of travelers. The first of the camps was set up along the beachfront. Daily, Beaumont watched this thaw; daily he saw Alexis strengthened. His time was running out.

One evening when Beaumont was walking back from the hospital, he spied two men standing atop the hillside. They waved him over.

It was Ramsay Crooks and Theodore Mathews.

"We've been star gazing, William," Mathews said.

"There it is." Crooks pointed. "Look, look there, gentlemen."

The three men stood in a line and watched the path of one and then another falling star.

"That's the seventh one this evening," Crooks explained. "It's been going on all week. Last night I saw three at one time. Has it never occurred to you gentlemen that we ought to be astronomers? That science came from wanderers and traders in the open spaces such as these?"

Mathews and Beaumont were equally entranced by the celestial show. They nodded in agreement.

"You fancy yourself an astronomer now, Ramsay?" Beaumont said.

"I tell you, William, I slept beneath these heavens for many nights when I was a younger man running furs for Mr. Astor. Hundreds. Perhaps a thousand. And only in these last few months have I thought of them anew. Look at what's about us. There are facts everywhere to be had. It was just the other day a question came to me. Although the Book of Genesis maintains that the stars are all set in the firmament to give light upon the earth, is it credible that the scheme of creation, with all its wondrous economy, should include globes far vaster than our own earth but destitute of life?"

Mathews spoke. "Those immense spheres are necessary conditions for the essential motions of the earth. Besides, their creation cost but the word of the omnipotent. Small price, I'd reckon."

"That's some strange currency you posit, Teddy. How, with the innumerable other suns and systems disposed irregularly at a distance, how is it that those stars give us no light and yet can still be the Creator's handiwork? Is the Creator wasteful with his handiwork? There must be others like us. How say you, Doctor?"

Beaumont chuckled. "A very great obstacle to science is an impatient proliferation of theory, leading to a hasty acceptance of dubious facts. Medicine's full of it, Ramsay."

"You think I play with theory?"

"Not at all, Ramsay. You're an empiricist if ever there was one."

Mathews spoke. "Mr. Crooks, you think there exist other planets with Christian men and the company?"

Crooks turned to face Mathews. "God made the Indian, did he not? He who smears himself with mud, cuts himself for penance and sees a deity in every plant, tree and stone. Those little brown ones your wife tries to teach to read. Give our Lord full faith and credit as a creator, Teddy. It took us how many centuries to be here as we are, and how many shall it take the savage to become as we are? How long will it take for one of those little ones to become president?" Crooks pointed to the smear of stars. "Is there not room for another planet of savages?"

Mathews smiled. "Tell that to the good reverend."

"Ah, science," Crooks mused. "Other works of genius are scarcely recognized now. Poetry is as dead as astrology, as religion. It's all for the women." He waved his right hand at the sky. "Names for each of these stars, their distances and positions, their intensities. The mind is overpowered in the attempt to amass such a vast storeroom of facts. A map for future travel to the next frontier. In these times, the deep searcher of the wonderful, of religion, the novelist, does not fear persecution, but rather *neglect*. He cannot interest the public. I tell this to my boys. This is the mechanical age. America is the country of the future, of beginnings, of projects, of vast designs and great expectations. The greatest triumphs of science are the most practical. This, gentlemen, is the age of steam."

They stood together, the three of them, for several minutes. Stars fell. The sound of a dog barking rose from the harbor, then ceased as abruptly as it had begun. Mathews shivered and tightened his coat collar.

"Doctor, you know my Abigail is among those who disapprove of Alexis and your charity for him, but I've long meant to tell you I admire what you've done for him. Your patience and your industriousness to heal the young man and make him a better man are exemplary. I admire you for that."

Beaumont had lowered his head as he listened to Mathews. "Thank you, Theodore," he said. "Such a sentiment fortifies my soul. I confess, it has been a rough winter."

"I'm sure my Abigail is wondering about me," Mathews stammered. "I should go, gentlemen. Good evening to you, Doctor, Mr. Crooks."

Theodore Mathews hurried off down the hill to the village.

Crooks spoke. "He's a queer young man. I'd fire him if I had the right man to replace him."

Beaumont and Ramsay watched Matthews disappear into the darkness.

"Ramsay, I've wanted to speak with you."

"I know," Crooks said simply.

"You know?"

"Go on, William. Speak to me."

"The thaw will soon commence, and with it I worry that the authorities will renew their pressure for Alexis to depart. Despite his innocence, despite his wound, despite all my charity. My private charity."

Crooks humphed.

"You seem, more so than the others, to recognize the folly in their ways. I've seen your smirks, your chuckles. Captain Pearce was irrational in his accusations that Alexis caused the stabbing or was some party to the event. And you as well know the value of an investment. I have invested too much in Alexis to simply cast him away in a boat to become a pauper or a freak in a circus show. I want to pay you for his indenture. It's forty dollars, is it not?"

"That's about right. Alexis St. Martin owes the American Fur Company forty dollars cash. Never mind the interest owed on the credit for the goods. That's probably another five dollars. It's a complicated system. Works to our advantage, if you gather the meaning of my words."

"Why don't I just pay you?"

Crooks stepped close enough to Beaumont that Beaumont could smell his sweet breath. The darkness seemed to lift. "Pay me the forty?"

"You erase your debt, he's free of the company, and when Captain Pearce comes griping to me about his drinking, we can just tell the captain to mind his soldiers. Pearce listens to you."

Crooks hesitated.

"I want peace among us all over this lad. Should I depart the island, given the company's reach and power, I could call on you if I should need help with Alexis."

Crooks mused over the proposition. The edges of his mouth were turned down, his lower lip puckered out. "You're a clever man, Doctor, a clever man. I do admire your devotion. What about thirty?"

"Ramsay?"

Crooks chuckled. "In silver."

"I've only paper notes, but I could get silver."

"Never the mind. Irony has never been your strength. Earnest, yes, all you Americans are that way, earnestness and pluck, but irony, no. Paper's fine, William. Just fine." Crooks shrugged his great shoulders. "Thirty, forty, what's ten dollars? Well, a lot to be sure. *A lot.* But the symbolism of the price overcame me for a moment."

Beaumont felt the grip of Crooks's right hand round his own. They shook.

"It's that wound, isn't it, William? The hole into the stomach. You've finally come to see its value. Or maybe you saw it that very first day, when you came back to the store to fetch him? You don't have to answer. I'm proud of you, William. Your earnestness and your pluck."

Crooks chuckled. He looked up at the sky, then looked back at Beaumont. "Your stellar aspirations. You can pay me when you have the money, and you can rest well assured. The company will watch over you and your digesting machine. He trusts you, you know. You're like his father, his savior."

{TWENTY-ONE}

THE DAY AFTER BEAUMONT PAID RAMSAY CROOKS the debt Alexis owed on his indenture, Elias sent for Alexis to meet him at the hospital. The three men stood in the space where Alexis had lived for a year and chatted about the many months of his slow recovery. Alexis lifted his shirt to show Elias his wound.

"You see," he smiled. "Healed up."

Elias leaned down, his hands upon his knees, to better inspect the scarred tissue and muscles, at the center of which was the hole sealed by the lid of pink flesh. He brushed the tip of his right index finger gently over the hole.

"If I'm not a Dutchman." He looked at Beaumont. "I'd never a thought."

Beaumont stood with his arms crossed upon his chest.

"It works handily to seal the cavity but yields readily to gentle digital pressure," he explained.

Elias whistled.

Alexis was still smiling. "Soon I will return to trapping."

"You can lower your shirt, Alexis," Beaumont said.

Alexis did as ordered.

The three men stood awkwardly like men at a dance without partners. Beaumont broke the silence. He reached and placed an arm over Alexis's shoulders.

"Alexis, why don't you step into my office for a minute? I thought it important we talk."

The two met sat across from each other at Beaumont's cluttered desk. Alexis kept to the edge of his chair; his hands gripped the seat as though he feared falling off. His black eyes surveyed the contents of the desk, the stacks of journals, papers and notebooks; pens and ink pots; animal bones. His gaze settled upon a jar full of green stones.

Beaumont took up the jar. "Those came from a banker in Plattsburgh. They're gallstones."

He held the jar out to Alexis.

The lad took it in hand and inspected it slowly, turning the jar over so the stones tumbled, and then he set it down.

"They come from the gallbladder, right below the liver. Interesting, are they not?"

Alexis nodded.

"Alexis, you have a, you have what I can only call a gift, a unique gift."

Alexis looked puzzled.

"What I mean is that you have something that you should share with others. That's what gifts are for."

"What should I share?"

Beaumont leaned forward over his arms. "I know you haven't considered it this way, but your wound. Your wound, Alexis. It's a kind of miracle."

Alexis nodded slowly.

"You have a wound that is without precedent, that is singular in the history of man. Your wound is a window into digestion. Through that hole the size of a half eagle you afford the opportunity for mankind to discover the secrets of one of the most essential parts of human health. Digestion."

Alexis pushed his hair back behind his ears. He blinked.

"You're precisely what Father Didier would pronounce a miracle."

"Father Didier," Alexis repeated.

"That's right. A miracle. God has given you a great gift that you can use for the betterment of mankind. Think about that, Alexis."

"God cured me."

"And he also left you with a hole in your side."

"I'm better."

"Better yes, but that hole remains, and that hole is a window to a world waiting to be discovered. God has given you a great opportunity to serve your fellow man. To make their lives better. A kind of noble calling, I think."

Alexis swallowed hard.

"Doctor, when can I go?"

"That is a fair question to which I'm obliged to answer fairly. The chores you do about the house are light and fair compensation, I should say, for your meals, the roof above your head, for your clothing. Mrs. Beaumont and I took you in out of the depth of our concern and charity for you. One year ago, when you were still here in this hospital recovering, the town wanted to cast you off in a bateau. I would not have that. It would have killed you. That's why Mrs. Beaumont and I took you in: so that you might live."

"I thank you for that, Doctor. But now I want to go back to fur trapping. I need to. I owe the company money."

Beaumont managed to smile. "You don't need to."

"Why?"

"Because you are no longer under the company's indenture."

"Why?"

"Ramsay Crooks sold it to me, Alexis. You're clean and whole. Your debt is forgiven."

Alexis straightened in his chair.

"So then I am bound to you?"

"Don't be silly, Alexis. I don't deal in papers that bind one man to another. You're a free man. As I said, your debt is paid. My appeal is to your reason, Alexis, to the better angels of your virtue."

"I can trap fur for whosoever I desire."

"You can, yes you can, but why would you do that when God has granted us the opportunity of a lifetime? A very wise and famous man once said 'What is serving God? 'Tis doing good to man.' The only men entitled to happiness are those who are useful."

Alexis stared at his hands.

"I'm to stay then?"

"That in exchange for room and board. But what I am talking about is the opportunity of your wound, to study inside it, to see how digestion proceeds in a healthy man such as you. I continue as your doctor, taking notes as I have done, gathering the gastric liquor as I have done, measuring the pace of digestion. You're well acquainted with all that. In my profession, Alexis, we have as a matter of principle that some good must come from the suffering we minister to. So others don't suffer. Otherwise men would remain as brutes do. Medicine is a science, and a doctor is a teacher. It's all very well to trap fur, but here is a chance to do something that will improve the lot of man. What do you say? In truth, this is no different really than what we've been doing since you moved in with Deborah and *petite* Sarah."

Beaumont cleared his throat and began to wag a carbon pencil between his fingers with such speed that the image of the thing became a blur. Alexis sat with his eyes closed and lips moving as if performing a complicated mental calculation. Beaumont set the pencil down neatly and folded the fingers of his two hands together into a tight braid.

"I'll pay you 15 dollars a month," Beaumont said. In one swift gesture, Beaumont rose from his chair to his full height. The scrape of the legs upon the floor was harsh. He extended his right hand to Alexis.

"Permit me to spare you the ciphering. That's 180 a year, Alexis. Fifteen paid in cash at the end of the month. With me covering your room and board, that is more than adequate, it's more like 20 dollars a month. Close to 200 or more a year."

Alexis opened his eyes and gazed at the right hand of his doctor. He crossed himself slowly, rose and extended his right hand across the desktop. They shook hands.

"So this then is my job, working for you with my stomach?"

Beaumont nodded. "That's a good lad."

IN MAY, A LETTER ARRIVED THAT bore Surgeon General Lovell's distinct and elegant cursive. Beaumont swallowed as he popped the red wax seal, the bits falling onto his desk like sugar candy. His hands trembled. This letter had the power to cleave time into time past and time future. Lovell could reject the case, reject the plans for experiments, or he could suggest the experiments be done by more qualified physicians. He could even order Alexis sent to Washington for his own study. Or he could give Beaumont his support and the freedom to study the man.

> Dear Doctor Beaumont,
>
> I have received your letter enclosing your valuable communication of the case of the wounded stomach. The cure is a full demonstration of the wonderful powers of Nature and highly creditable to yourself. Agreeable to your suggestion, I shall send it to the Medical Recorder for publication.
>
> I will endeavor to send you some books of experiments on the gastric liquor, which will be somewhat of a guide to you in making your observations, which may be done with perfect ease and safety. It is stated, for example, that if several articles of food be taken into the stomach, that it would digest all of one kind first, then all of a second, and so on, and that this is the cause of the bad effects of a variety of food at the same meal.
>
> Suppose a man eat beef, potatoes, fish, cabbage and pudding. It is expected that he will first digest all the beef, the others in the meantime remaining untouched. Then all of the pudding, then all the potatoes, and lastly the cabbage.
>
> Now, it is thought that if he eat a dozen articles, by the time the stomach has disposed of eight or ten, it will become exhausted, and the rest will be left to ferment and produce indigestion and its consequent evils. Could you make an experiment to ascertain this, and also the digestibility of various articles?
>
> This alone would afford a most valuable paper for publication. I should be happy to receive an account of any experiments or observations you may make, and they will not doubt be very acceptable to the public.
>
> Yours truly,
> Surgeon General Joseph Lovell

Two days later, an inspired Dr. William Beaumont sat with knife and cutting board at the kitchen table. He prepared pieces of high-seasoned beef, raw salted fat pork, raw salted lean beef, boiled salted beef, bread and a bunch of raw cabbage. Each he cut to weigh about two drachms, making his best estimate of the weight. The cabbage he sliced into finger-length strips. He uncoiled a length of silk string, some two feet he estimated from the tip of his middle finger to his elbow, cut it, and secured the seasoned beef to the end, measured the distance of his forefinger along the string and there secured the piece of pork and so on until he had secured each piece of food in a kind of chain. Then he cut the excess of the string.

He admired the precision of his work. The thing turned clockwise, stopped, then turned counterclockwise.

Around noon, Alexis stepped indoors from his chores. The past several days had been unusually hot and dry. The air was heavy and still. Horses had kicked up dust that lingered in the air like smoke. Men moved slowly and napped at noon beneath shade trees.

Alexis was barefoot and dressed in a close-fitting pair of breeches and a sleeveless gray shirt damp with sweat at his chest and armpits. He had washed his face in the rain barrel, and his damp hair was slicked back. He took up the water pitcher, filled his wooden cup and took a great drink, poured himself another drink, then eased himself into his customary place at the table.

There were no platters on the table.

"Am I late?"

Beaumont was closing up the ice chest, from which he was removing a porcelain basin containing the articles of food for the experiment.

"No, no, not at all. Mrs. Beaumont is out with the children for the day. It's Monday. Washing day. They should return after noon, but I've got your supper ready. It's a full meal."

Beaumont stood in his shirtsleeves. He held the basin in one arm and gestured to it with the other. "The only difference—and a slight difference at that—is that I'll put it in as I've done before, through the hole to your stomach. I think you'll like it. A meal of seasoned beef, fat pork, some salted beef, bread, of course, and some cabbage. You take that in, go back to work, and I'll check on the progress of your digestion. All of it as we've done before many times, only this time the circumstances are more controlled."

Alexis looked at Beaumont. "What if I still have hunger?"

"By the evening meal you'll be set to eat more. You had a thorough breakfast this morning. Four, perhaps five hours, is all I'd think."

Alexis drained his cup.

Beaumont gestured to the door to Alexis's room. "So then," he announced. "Step into your room. It'll just take a moment, and then you're back to work."

Alexis lay on his cot with his arms folded behind his head and his legs straight and uncrossed. The two men had discovered that when Alexis was stretched out in this position it eased the opening of the flap of gastric tissue that secured the hole closed. Beaumont slid the length of his index finger into the hole. The cavity was warm and moist and entirely empty. He removed the cloth from the basin wherein he kept the garland of food and held it up so its contents uncoiled. He eased it into the hole. Alexis winced as it crossed the tender cuticle. A good twelve inches of string remained outside the aperture, and this Beaumont coiled securely about a four-inch, flat piece of polished mahogany, curved so that it sat firmly against the wound and shaped to assure it could not enter the hole.

He took note of the time.

Alexis looked down at the piece of mahogany.

"That secures the silk thread upon which are the articles of food you're digesting for supper." Beaumont produced a roll of bandages. "Now then, raise up your arms. You know the drill."

He covered the wound with a simple crossing of bandages.

"Good then. I'll have a look in an hour. Here you are."

He held out Alexis's shirt.

As Alexis swept, Beaumont took up his notebook and carbon. He began to write but then he stopped. He sat for a moment, and then he took out the letter from Lovell and reread it. *This alone would afford a most valuable paper for publication.* First he would publish his case report, then his study of the digestibility of multiple articles of alimentation. In just one year, his two papers would enter his name into the medical literature. First fame. Fortune would follow.

One hour later, Alexis lay upon his back in the customary position, and Beaumont withdrew the string, taking care to minimize the discomfort as the articles passed over the tender cuticle. He laid the length of string out carefully on a towel. The cabbage and bread were half digested. The pieces of meat slightly were gray but otherwise unchanged. He returned the food parts into the stomach.

He recorded his observations, and beneath them he made notes. The facts were opposite to his expectations. The cabbage should be digested last, but it was digesting first. The beef should digest first, but it remained essentially undigested.

When the clock struck two, he withdrew the string again. The cabbage, bread, pork and boiled beef were all gone from the string. The high-seasoned beef and raw salted lean beef remained very little affected by the digestion. He returned them into the stomach. His observations upset the conventional expectations. *Did I chop the cabbage too finely?* he wrote. He took up his copy of Antiquel's history, opened it without care and tried to read as he waited for the third hour.

"Doctor, I am not well."

Alexis stood before Beaumont. His face was pale, and he held his right hand over his stomach.

"I am sick at the stomach and the head."

Beaumont snapped the book closed.

"On to your cot."

"I feel sick."

"Just lie down as usual."

The two pieces of beef were nearly in the same condition as when he had last examined them. He leaned closer to the gastric cavity and sniffed. He sniffed again. The odor was rancid and sharp, and the surface of the gastric tissue bore a few tiny white papules. He measured Alexis's pulse. Regular but bounding. He ran the back of his hand over his forehead and the skin of his chest. Warm and dry. The phenomena of fever, but he was not feverish.

"How do you feel now?"

Alexis shook his head.

"How's your stomach?"

Alexis grimaced and shook his head again. "Not good," he muttered.

"Don't fret. It's minor venous congestion."

Alexis moaned as he drew his skinny legs up to his chest. Beaumont sat back on his chair and observed the lad. The bottoms of his feet were dark and calloused. He looked down at the two pieces of undigested beef. The facts made no sense. To be sure, the multiple items of aliment had led to indigestion, but the pace and order of digestion was not as he had expected. He had suspended beef, raw and cooked, into the cavity many times before, and they were always digested within two hours. He had sampled meals of meat and vegetable with a siphon and seen the slow pace of vegetable matter.

"How are you?"

Alexis did not open his eyes.

"Alexis?"

"My head."

"Yes?"

"My stomach."

Beaumont measured Alexis's pulse. Without change.

"Just rest there as you are. You'll mend soon."

"I could puke."

"Don't try. There's nothing there."

Beaumont stepped into the kitchen and gazed at his notebook wherein he simply wrote, *beef remains undigested, complains of distress at stomach and head & costiveness,* and then he shut the notebook.

"What am I doing?"

IN THE EVENING, a whitish coating had developed over Alexis's tongue, his pulse was depressed, and Beaumont found numerous pustules spread over the stomach's surface. The water Alexis passed was dark and foul smelling. After Beaumont emptied the chamber pot in the bucket beside the shed, he stood for some time in his yard, gazing at the night sky. How odd that a man like Ramsay Crooks wished to make a study of the stars when there was so much to discover here on earth. He whistled for Rex, but the dog did not come. He had not seen the dog for several days. Weeks even.

He considered the experiment again and yet again. Perhaps he had demonstrated that a stomach filled with multiple items of aliment will exhaust itself, and some items will be retained and ferment. The bread was stale and so porous as to readily admit the gastric juice and fall off the string. The cabbage was chopped too fine. But why the meat, and only some of the meat, why did it resist the powers of the gastric juice?

When he returned inside, Deborah was seated at her dressing table brushing out her hair. "What's wrong with Alexis?"

"Some distress at his stomach and head. It'll mend."

She continued brushing her hair.

"Is he ill?"

Beaumont shook his head. "Simply recovering from too much variety of food. Cabbage, bread, beef boiled, à la mode and raw, and salted fat pork."

"That's quite a supper, even for a laborer."

Beaumont explained the day's experiment to his wife while she completed her toilet. When he finished, they were lying side by side in the darkness. She yawned. Washing day exhausted her. She did not speak for some time, and when she did, her voice was small and soft, like drizzle on leaves.

"What will you report to Dr. Lovell?"

He considered her question. "Honestly, I think my results are important from the pathologic point of view. They confirm the common opinion that undigested aliment retained in the stomach produces all the phenomena of fever. It's clear evidence of the danger of excess in aliment."

"I suppose then you can write him about that and see what he has to surmise."

"Perhaps. But I think it wise to try some other experiments prior to sending a report. That was just the first, and tentative as well. It raises as many questions as it answers. But I have written to Lovell to request a transfer and review of my rank. We've been here now five years. It's high time I have my choice of another fort and promotion to surgeon."

"Yes," she said. Her voice was thick and heavy with sleep.

"As soon as next spring, perhaps Fort Howard. Or even Plattsburgh. Or St. Louis. Wouldn't that be grand?"

It would be grand. Any of those places would be grand. But as he was talking about their hope for the future, he was thinking about his past, about his apprentice years when he slept in a low-ceilinged loft above the kitchen while Dr. Chandler lay beside his golden-haired wife in a room of their own. Beaumont rose early, before the rest of the household. He sat on the edge of a milking stool, his thin frame curled close over the low pine table that was wedged beside his narrow and lonely bed. A circle of candle-light illuminated his medical text's soft pages, and the sand on the kitchen floor glowed pale like the lonely moonscape. He copied passages into note-books, recorded cases, recited treatments. His cold fingers were stained with ink and his nails bitten to their bloody quick. He worked hard with the belief that his labor would one day free him of poverty and his humble origins. And now, some fifteen years later, he was back at that table.

{TWENTY-THREE}

THE NEXT MORNING, ALEXIS STILL LAY with his legs curled up to his chest and complained about his stomach and head. Beaumont inserted a half a dozen calomel pills directly into the gastric cavity. Within three hours, these induced a brisk, cathartic response, and by the afternoon, Alexis had recovered. Following a supper of cold beef, potatoes and pudding, he performed his usual chores.

In the days following the first experiment, a keen energy possessed Beaumont. He rose early. He retired late. He kept reaching for his notebook to jot an idea, or if the notebook was not handy, any odd scrap of paper. He was planning to prove the chemical nature of digestion. The stomach was not a grinding machine or a fermenting vat. Gastric juice was not inert. He'd tasted its acrid, sharp flavor many times. He'd even put a few drops on a cut along his forearm and felt its sting. It was a chemical. What he needed was to prove it through a series of experiments varying the articles of aliment and the conditions of digestion.

The necessary test was to isolate the action of the juice upon aliment in conditions without the grinding and churning and the possibility of fermentation. The solution came to him as he stood outside the blacksmith's shop watching the sweating man heft a stone jar of molten iron from a fire kept red and furious by his two sons' rhythmic pumping of the bellows.

The solution was heat. The chemicals he had tasted in the juice required heat to react. He knew that proper temperature from previous observations of Alexis's stomach. One hundred degrees on his Fahrenheit thermometer. But how to make the heat steady and general around the vial of juice so as to mimic the stomach's surrounding warmth? This question the blacksmith answered. A sand bath.

Beaumont was pleased with himself. A silk thread he'd divined from watching soldiers feed a length of it to a goat, then slowly pull it out. The gum elastic tube to extract gastric liquor he'd discovered while watching a child drink sweetened tea. And now a blacksmith's sand bath. He had solved his heat problem. He would nestle the vial into a basin filled with dry sand of constant and regular granularity and place that basin upon a fire. The caloric action would travel uniformly through the sand and surround the vial like the warm flesh of a man's innards.

LATE ONE SUNDAY MORNING following the Reverend James's service, Beaumont excused himself from conversation with Abigail and Theodore Mathews and hurried home to set up his sand bath and wait for Alexis's return from Father Didier's chapel among the tents along the beachfront. Didier had a strange burlesque ritual that ended with serving wine and bread he claimed to transform into Jesus Christ's blood and body, but only to those who had fasted. A small amount of wine and bread would rapidly digest. The cavity would be entirely empty and prepared for his experiment.

And it was.

"Very simple plan here, Alexis. I want to take the measure of temperature in here and then draw off some of the liquor. I'll give you a piece of cooked beef, a small piece, and suspend it as I have done before. You should digest that within an hour or two, and then we'll have dinner."

"May I walk about?"

"Just here in the house."

Alexis folded his arms behind his head and stared up at the ceiling as Beaumont took up his Fahrenheit thermometer from its felt-lined case. He wiped the length of it with a cotton cloth he kept expressly for this purpose, then slowly inserted the thermometer into the cavity. He marked the top of the column with ink, and then he withdrew it and placed it upon the ruler. The ink mark read one hundred degrees. He wiped the column carefully, set it into its case and took up his gum elastic tube.

"Now then, onto your left side." He guided Alexis with his hands. "There now. The elastic tube."

Alexis let out a small whimper.

"Tell me if the sinking feeling happens."

Beaumont carefully inserted the tube, taking care not to rub the tender cuticle of the hole's margin.

"Really, Alexis, this is minor," he remarked. "Remember that first autumn after the shooting? When the wound started expelling pieces of shot and clothing? You once coughed up a button."

Alexis nodded.

Within two minutes the slow trickle of juice began to flow. Beaumont gently moved the tube back and forth, in and out, as the trickle continued. After a few minutes Alexis moaned. He told the lad to bear with him, and in another minute he withdrew the tube. The vial contained some three ounces of clear gastric juice.

"Stay please, lad."

Beaumont stepped quickly to the kitchen hearth. He set a piece of boiled and recently salted beef into the vial, corked the vial tight and nestled it into the sand bath as far as the cork. Then he returned to Alexis, who lay with one leg flexed and rocking slowly to and fro, the other stretched out.

"Now then," Beaumont said, and he straightened out Alexis's leg. He eased his forefinger into the cavity, then followed this with a piece cut from the same beef, precisely the same size and shape, tied neatly as a gift box with a piece of silk thread. As before, he let the piece fall into the cavity, let the flap of tissue close and wrapped the length of string outside the cavity around the curved mahogany piece.

"That's all. Why don't you put on your shirt, and we can have look in about an hour? Alexis?"

"Maybe I just lie here."

He patted Alexis's thigh. "Whatever you wish. I shall be out in the kitchen."

He checked the vial in the sand bath regularly. It was evident after forty minutes that digestion had commenced over the surface of the beef. After ten more minutes the fluid had become quite opaque and cloudy. He had to uncork the vial to inspect the beef. Its surface was quite loose.

When Beaumont returned to inspect the gastric digestion of the beef, he found Alexis lying upon his side running his index finger slowly along the seams of the wall. Beaumont ordered him onto his back and withdrew the string. The beef was as much affected by digestion as that in the vial. He leaned close to the aperture and sniffed. The smell was clean. Not putrid. The tissue of the gastric lining was pink and glistening. He returned the beef to the cavity.

One hour later, the muscular fibers of the beef in the vial were reduced to small, loose, unconnected shreds. He took a few fibers into the palm of his hand: they were tender and soft. He returned them to the vial and corked it.

When Beaumont withdrew the string from Alexis's cavity, all that remained were the two loops that had once held the beef snug like some queer hangman's double noose.

These were glorious proofs that the process of digestion was not simply grinding and certainly not fermentation or putrefaction. It was chemical. And boiled beef was just the first test. There were other foods: salted beef, beef à la mode, roasted beef, chicken, both boiled and roasted, venison, salted cod and a variety of vegetables as well. Milk and eggs. Certainly spirituous liquors too.

{TWENTY-FOUR}

HE WOULD HAVE DONE MORE EXPERIMENTS. He had sketched out detailed plans to observe the temperature of the stomach and regularly sample the chyme and its temperature. But in that first week of June he received a letter announcing that an inspector from the surgeons' corps was making the rounds of the Northern territories. Dr. Lyman Foote would arrive within the month.

Elias and he prepared the hospital. They used pine tar to caulk the seams and replaced several rotting floorboards. Beaumont convinced the quartermaster to give him two new cots to replace those that were broken beyond repair. They inventoried their supplies, swept out all the cabinets, dusted all their bottles and jars and used this occasion to prepare a fresh set of medicinals from the garden.

Dr. Lyman Foote arrived midday aboard the regal steamship *Saratoga*. Surgeon in the U.S. Army, Fellow of the College of Physicians of Philadelphia, and Correspondent of the Lyceum of Natural History, New York, he was nearing the end of his four-month tour inspecting the garrison hospitals of the Northern territories. Authorized by Congress and appointed by his friend and Harvard classmate Surgeon General Joseph Lovell, he traveled with an aide, a deferential corporal, pox marked and with crooked yellowed teeth, who lugged along a much-used lap desk.

ON THE EVENING OF FOOTE'S ARRIVAL, Captain Pearce hosted a dinner in his honor. The officers, officials of the company, village leaders and Foote assembled in the officers' mess. Soldiers butlered platters of drinks and savories. When the room grew noisy and hot, the windows were flung open, and more bottles were decanted. Moths fluttered across the ceiling, and a full moon illuminated the room. The fort glowed like a phosphorescent castle.

After more than an hour of conversation fueled by drinks and food, the men were garrulous and at ease in conversation and laughter. It took several minutes to get them to settle at the long table. Once seated, order was briefly restored when Captain Pearce tapped his knife blade gently upon his claret glass.

"Reverend James," he intoned.

The reverend scratched his arms and placed his thin hands together. Every man bowed his head.

"Dear Lord, bless this gathering of your humble servants and the journey of our guest, Dr. Foote."

When the reverend finished, Pearce snapped his chin up, thanked the reverend briskly and raised his claret glass.

"Gentlemen, let me commence with the first toast of the evening. To the United States Army and to our distinguished guest, Surgeon Hyman Flute."

Some swilled. Others sipped carefully.

There were courses of meats, fishes and vegetables. A fresh-slaughtered steer in a wild mushroom gravy, roasted guinea fowl glazed with citrus and molasses, varieties of squash baked with honey and butter, white potatoes mashed with chestnuts, cabbages, three kinds of wine and lake trout caught that very afternoon in Mackinac harbor.

Several of the guests queried Foote about steamship travel. Others joined in with their opinions on the future of transport in America. One wondered if there were any new inventions to create. Still another said he had heard of steamships that could travel on land.

As Foote was slicing a squash into neat pieces, he asked those near him, "I understand you maintain a garden at this fort?"

The assembly looked to Pearce.

"We do," Pearce announced.

"Excellent," said Foote. He continued chewing. "Secretary of War Calhoun shares our view that a soldier's diet needs a proper balance of vegetables as well as legumes. Simply subsisting on fried meats and bread debilitates a man's constitution."

Pearce was smiling. "We've heard."

"What about the whiskey ration?" asked Hardage Thompson.

Foote gestured with his fork. "That's next. Though don't press me for the details, as I don't have them. I can assure you that there is a general recognition among the command that ardent spirits are not a necessary part of the ration, that it is the cause of a general debilitation of the soldier's constitution. Reputation, honor, health and even life are sacrificed to obtain the inebriating draught."

Several of the guests began remarking on the subject of the whiskey ration, but they stopped when Pearce spoke up.

"What about fighting? What's the talk among the command about that?"

"I beg your pardon, Captain?"

Pearce was red faced, and the hair at his temples was damp with sweat. "Best way to maintain the Constitution, capital *C* on that too, is to keep an army fighting. The Sioux, the Fox, the Creek, Canada, La Republica de Mexico. Why isn't this army fighting?"

Foote was visibly uncomfortable. "You've asked the wrong man, Captain. That's a query best put to Secretary Calhoun, I should think."

Pearce drained his glass and tapped its rim with his forefinger. A waiter stepped close with a decanter and began to refill it. Pearce watched the red wine rise to the rim. Then he looked at Foote.

"I know," he said dully. "I'll leave you all to your vegetables." He gestured to Theodore Mathews. "You there, Teddy, why don't you pass that platter of stewed cabbage to our guest?"

By the hour when the pudding laced with both white and red raisins was sent round, the rules of the officers' mess had been broken, and several officers were given the punishment of having to bring a bottle to the next mess, one man for spilling his wine on the table, two for leaving the table to void and a third who garbled his remarks on the report of an uprising among the Fox Indians near Fort Crawford. Theodore Mathews was heavy lidded and staring at his plate.

Captain Pearce was animated, praising General Jackson's battles against the Seminole Indians and his rule of the Florida territory. Russell Stuart, the Indian agent, advanced the thesis that the Seminoles were among the least civilized of the Indians, owing to their tropical conditions. They seemed centuries behind the Indians of the Plains, who had built villages and farms.

"Interbreeding with the African slave runaways did not help," he asserted. "History shows us the pace of civilization. The nomad of the desert, the heathen of the Levant. Civilization comes slowly to those who wander, and the climate plays no small role in that."

Pearce looked to others at the table. "Doctor," he said.

Both Foote and Beaumont looked to Pearce.

"You there." Pearce gestured to Foote. "Yes, you. Flute. Have you seen our good Dr. Beaumont's Frenchman with the bunghole in his side?"

Foote looked confused. "I'm sorry?" He was visibly tired. The pearl buttons of his vest strained, and his cravat was loosened and askew.

"He's got a wounded voyageur with a lid on his stomach. You haven't told our guest of your Frenchman, Dr. Beaumont?"

Beaumont cleared his throat. "Dr. Foote arrived just this afternoon, Captain. He's not had the opportunity to begin his inspection."

"What's this?" Foote asked Beaumont.

Pearce was animated. "It's fantastic, Doctor. A preternatural wonder." He looked about the table. "Isn't it, Russell? Hardage? Teddy?"

The men said nothing. Beaumont searched the table for Ramsay Crooks. He was gone.

Pearce carried on.

"The man was good for dead. Dead, I tell you, but our Dr. Beaumont saved his life. Shotgun blast to his left side, right here." Pearce placed his hand over the spot and made the sound of the discharge. "Right here, and it was a mess of food about, not to mention the blood and such. I saw living and breathing lung. Looked just like a turkey's egg. Days to follow they were picking out shot from the wall. And that was what, some two, three years ago, and now the lad walks about, eats and drinks, does he drink, and works as a common servant here for the doctor. How's that for charity?"

"A lid?" Foote asked.

"A lid," Pearce bellowed as he flapped his hand up and down as if to demonstrate the action. "He's got some sort of lid right into his stomach. Blows out gas, I'd bet."

Foote looked to Beaumont. "Pray tell?"

Beaumont cleared his throat. "The captain has well summarized the essential details," he said. "Tomorrow you will see Alexis, that's his name. I shall explain the particulars of the case then. Surgeon General Lovell has been well apprised, and I have submitted a report to the *Medical Recorder*."

"But a lid?"

"A gastrocutaneous fistula developed, and in time a fold of tissue has come to act as a sort of valve to prevent egress of the contents."

"And yet you can open it?" Foote asked.

The soldiers, even some of the waiters and the barefoot boy with the water pitcher, were looking to Beaumont.

"It can be opened, yes. I'll show you tomorrow."

Foote's attention was thoroughly restored. "And once opened, you have a kind of window into the process of digestion, correct? He's been alive for some two years now? He must have normal digestion, and yet, and yet, with the passage of air into the cavity that would limit the degree of fermentation."

Beaumont simply nodded.

Pearce interrupted. "Bring him here, why not? Right here."

"Captain?" Beaumont looked visibly distressed.

Pearce thumped the tabletop with his knuckles. "Bring. Him. Here. *Here*. There's plenty for him to eat. By God, look at that cheese." He gestured to a plate with three rounds of cheese. "Why wait until the morrow to show our distinguished guest?" he insisted. "You've never made a proper display of the man, after all we've done for him. He's been a bit of a piece, I assure you, Dr. Flute. Last season there was a riot on the beach after he won a drinking bet. Poured it down and poured it out. Oh, how clever are those Frenchies."

Pearce rotated in his chair. He spied his corporal in the shadows beside the mantle.

"Corporal, hurry over to the Beaumonts' cottage and fetch the Frenchman. Tell him he has a personal invitation from Captain Isaiah Ignatius Pearce to the officers' banquet." Pearce held his right forefinger aloft. "A personal invitation."

Beaumont spoke up.

"Captain, I should think the man is retired by now. Moreover, the inspection of his wound is a medical matter, not something for an officers' mess entertainment."

Foote was nodding in agreement.

The corporal stood still and wide-eyed. He looked to the doctors. Then he looked to Pearce, who gestured casually to the corporal as he gazed at Beaumont and said with a delicate menace, "Why don't we let the lad decide that, Doctor? He's a free man, is he not? Corporal," he barked, "you have your orders."

Beaumont sat rigid.

"Captain, my wife and children. They're likely asleep."

"A doctor's wife should be well accustomed to interruptions."

CIGARS AND A WICK WERE PASSED and the brandies brought forth. Soon the room was a haze of blue smoke, and the assembly began to rise from the table. Pearce drained his glass and walked slowly to the window with a view to the lake. The dock was empty, the steamship having departed early in the evening.

Foote leaned close to Beaumont. "Really, Doctor, this can wait until tomorrow. Now's not the proper time for an examination of any man. I shall talk with the captain."

Foote began to rise from his chair, but Beaumont checked him as he shook his head. "Don't. Not when he's in this sort of state. I assure you, I have every intention of showing you the case and the experiments I've undertaken." He leaned close to the physician's ear. "I've begun to establish the chemical nature of digestion."

"Chemical?"

"Yes. Chemical. Not a fermenting vat, not a grinding device, but a chemical process."

Beaumont explained his experiments. He concluded by describing the vial of whey-colored gastric juice. "Some three weeks later, and it retains its sweet aroma. Not even a whiff of putrefaction, and except for gentle agitation, it was not subjected to the slightest grinding."

Foote was silent for a moment. "Spallanzani has a theory of chemical digestion."

"And Beaumont has proved it," Beaumont announced.

In the months and years that followed this conversation, Beaumont would recall their exchange and recoil with shame over his pride. One experiment proved little. Dr. Lyman Foote knew that as well as any educated man. And yet he spoke those words. *Beaumont has proved it.*

The corporal returned alone. He whispered to Pearce, who shrugged and nodded. The corporal turned quickly on his heel. As he was crossing the room, Beaumont caught his eye. The corporal stepped close to Beaumont.

"He wasn't at home, sir," he whispered.

It was past midnight when Beaumont tapped a knuckle sharply on the door to Alexis's room. No answer came. He eased the door open.

"Alexis." He stood at the threshold to let his eyes adjust to the darkness. The space felt empty, cold.

A voice whispered behind him. "William?"

Deborah reached for his shoulder but then set her hand down. "William, what's wrong? There was a soldier here asking for Alexis."

"And?"

"I told him he wasn't here."

Beaumont stepped into the small room. The bed was empty. He slapped the thing.

"William, what's happening?"

He sat heavily on the edge of the narrow bed, his head in his hands.

"I don't know."

"Why did a soldier come for him?" Her voice was scared.

"Pearce," he spat. "Pearce was drunk. He wanted him to come to the dinner, to have me show Alexis off. Show him off. Can you fathom that?"

She held out her hand to her husband. "Come to bed, William."

"I'll be back within the hour."

"Where are you going?"

"What do you think, woman? To find him."

"William, it's late. Late. Please," she begged. "He's a young man, and it's a full moon. He could be anywhere among the tents along the lakeshore, in the barracks, in the woods. You'll not find him."

Beaumont just stood still before his wife.

"Just come to bed," she pleaded.

DEPTH OF DAWN. Beaumont did not stop running until he reached the water's edge. His chest ached, and his legs burned. There were a few Indians and voyageurs moving slowly among the tents and lean-tos. They stared at Beaumont as he stood heaving at the water's edge, his shirttails loose. A corncob, a few animal bones, bits of firewood and a green bottle rolled in the gentle lapping of the waves. The dock was empty. The steamship had departed in the early evening.

He turned. Two women wrapped in blankets squatted before a low cooking fire. One of them was old and toothless and gray. The other might have been her daughter. A small boy stood between them. He was dressed only in a pair of ragged buckskin trousers tied with a piece of rope, and he fingered his protuberant navel. His face was blemished with lesions. The three of them stared at him with unblinking ebony eyes. The old woman spoke in a guttural tongue.

"Well," he asked them, "I don't suppose you know where he is?"

The boy hurried into the tent.

Beaumont spat. He punched the air. He kicked the earth. He kicked it again so hard he nearly fell on his rump. Several soldiers were walking toward him. Major Hardage Thompson was in the lead. When they reached Beaumont, the major simply stood. He was not yet dressed for morning parade. The breeze tossed his thin gray hair.

Beaumont held out a folded paper. "He left this," he said plainly.

Thompson unfolded it. One edge was jagged, as though it had been torn to fashion a puzzle piece. He looked at the paper, and then he looked at Beaumont.

"It's his half of his indenture agreement with the company." Beaumont explained. "That's all he left. That and two vials."

PART 2

The Only Men Entitled to Happiness

TWENTY-FIVE

THE WINTER OF 1824 BEGAN with stories of hostile Indian activity in the territories around the northern waters of the Mississippi River. The Sioux, Sauk, Winnebago and Fox Indians were disputing their boundaries. The agents of the Department of Indian Affairs paid out more and more presents and compensations, but the disagreements only intensified.

In time, anger among the tribes spilled over to the whites. In the early spring of 1825, at the end of maple-syrup-making season, the Methode family did not return to the village of Prairie du Chien on the banks of the Mississippi River in Wisconsin. A search party found them murdered and scalped in their camp near Painted Rock Creek. Mother, father, three children and dog. The camp was burned, the packed snow crimson.

The governors of Illinois, Wisconsin and Michigan threatened to call up their militias. The army began to move troops and supplies about the Northern territories. Captain Pearce was assigned the command of Fort Snelling, but before he could depart for this duty, his aide found him dead at his desk. A bullet wound to his forehead. The implements of his gun-cleaning equipment were scattered; the whiskey bottle was empty. Brevet Major Hardage Thompson was transferred to Fort Edwards, and Surgeon General Lovell ordered Beaumont to assist in outfitting the hospitals of the Great Lakes region. His skills from the War of 1812 were most valued.

When the order arrived, Deborah had begged her husband to leave the army and set up a private practice in St. Louis. She dreaded life on the road, the weeks of hot and dusty travel, the long days rocking in crowded, damp boats, living out of trunks.

He rejected her plea. He told her that with the long shadow of the Griswold affair still darkening his name and his promotion to surgeon uncertain, to quit was to concede failure and surrender his reputation. Lovell needed him, and this service might restore his reputation.

In time, they came to enjoy the journey. They wound through miles of woods and passed apple orchards heavy with fruit. They traveled between walls described by fields of tall corn or hay. They crossed narrow rivers drawn down by summer's heat, trout visible in the clear pools, their fins like tiny Japanese silk fans. They yielded the way for teamsters who drove wagons filled with sacks of grain and lumber.

They rested beneath shade trees beside ponds. Beaumont carried Sarah piggyback and swung her round in fields of poppies and lupine. The two of them chased spooked rabbits. She delighted at the panicked shrieks of flushed quail. They watched thunderstorms gather in the afternoon, and at night, heat lightning cast the trees in silhouette. Sarah kept up a steady chatter of questions, and he obliged them with patient answers.

They dined at inns where the clientele of well-to-do farmers clapped their thick hands as their wives sang songs in Old German. They watched children dance hand-in-hand in counter-turning circles. They fed Sarah her first peach, the golden juice dribbling off her chin. Several nights, they slept beneath a canvas tarp; little Sarah lay between them whimpering and kicking in her dreams like a puppy.

The infant William had died the previous winter of fever that struck him on a Monday like a dart. Beaumont rubbed the child with spirits of camphor, bled him from a tiny vein, but by Wednesday the child would not take to his mother's breast, and around noon on Friday, just four weeks after his first birthday, the boy took his last breath in his mother's arms.

In time, their grief became bearable. The travels helped. But a different grief still preoccupied him: his loss of Alexis St. Martin. The savor of the days of experiments was gone. All that remained was a bitter anger. Beaumont calculated that by the day Alexis fled, he had spent some 360 dollars on his ungrateful Frenchman. He had spent hundreds of hours, hours when he could have been earning income. He came to despise the experiments, and he shuddered with shame over his dreams. He cringed when he recalled again and yet again his miscalculations with Alexis.

Even the case report, the one return upon his investment, taunted him. It was published in January 1825, in the *Medical Recorder,* but under the name of Dr. Joseph Lovell, Washington City. Five months later, a correction appeared: *The case of the fur trapper with a gastric fistula was reported by Dr. William Beaumont, Mackinac Island in the Michigan Territory.* The correction was small consolation. He was forced to maintain his place in Medicine's order. The credit went to the Harvard-trained physician.

He found solace writing in his notebook. His pen worked like a scalpel; his words were a surgery cutting away his grief and frustration.

Why will you not accept your lot in life as your brothers, as your father, do? You could have all you have—your wife, your child, your small fortune, your commission in the army—you could have all you have and yet be content.

One morning, after several miles of silent travel along a misty road, as they ate apple slices while Sarah slept in her mother's arms, Deborah turned to her husband, smiled and kissed his cheek.

"'Tis a gift to be simple," she said.

He smiled, and then he returned her kiss on her lips. "Indeed it is."

BY FALL, THE RUMORS OF WAR had vanished. A Great Council of all the tribes, the Indian agents and the army drew up new borders and promised generous compensations to respect these borders. The chiefs smoked the peace pipe and buried the war tomahawk with a promise never to raise it again as long as the waters of the Mississippi ran free. William, Deborah and Sarah Beaumont settled into the surgeon's quarters at Fort Howard, on the banks of the Fox River in Green Bay, Wisconsin. Within a month William Beaumont, MD, was promoted to surgeon in the U.S. Army.

Finally, he could start his life and his career anew.

He set to his work with the zeal of his youth. He and Deborah attended dinner parties and dances in the society of officers and agents of the American Fur Company. The wives organized a chorus and a literary salon. The officers performed theatricals in the mess hall. By spring, Sarah could sing her alphabet, Beaumont had purchased a forty-acre lot along the Fox River, and Deborah had given birth to a girl they named Lucretia.

A mild winter followed by a dry spring was conducive to the health of the populace, but in the summer, two weeks of rains swelled the river and flooded the swamps into waist-deep ponds. The waters spread over the lowlands. The hay fields were flooded, and when the river receded, stagnant pools and shallow ponds remained. Green frogs appeared from the muck, and within a week, the still water turned brown, bubbles rose and the swamp fevers began. They did not cease until the first frost.

Beaumont began drafting notes for an article on the nature and character of the intermittent fevers of the Fox River Valley. His notebooks, though, less and less preoccupied him. In time, he put them away. Entire months passed without a thought of Alexis, and when some event kindled a memory, when he read a report of a fascinating surgical case, the memory of his ambition was like the recollection of romantic desire. Distant, small and fading.

He had decided there was neither pleasure nor profit to be had by writings and scientific experiment. His pleasure was his growing family, and his profit was in the practice of medicine, and investment in land. In the past year, he had befriended Hector Berny, the land agent, and with Berny's sagacious advice, he had purchased three contiguous parcels of land in Green Bay, now 120 acres total, suitable for farming, proximal to the river for trade, but well above the floodplain. Beaumont's Saturday-afternoon tally of his wealth made him content. Deborah was right. It was a gift to be simple and to live in the corruptions of neither poverty nor wealth, but solidly in the middle. He planned to resign from the army and set up a private practice in St. Louis.

On the afternoon of the 17th of August, 1827, the corporal in charge of the mails delivered Beaumont a letter whose return address bore the name

Theodore Mathews, Agent of the American Fur Company, Sackett's Harbor, New York.

15 July 1827
Dear Dr. Beaumont,

I trust this letter finds you and your family well & happy and settled among good friends. Abigail and I speak frequently & fondly of those pleasant years of convivial sociability on Mackinac Island among our little Island Village. I remain under the employment of the Company and obtained promotion to agent; gone are my shop keeper days. The fur trade remains prosperous though talk is that its Grand Days are fading; pelts are not as readily plentiful & competition harries us & fashion shifts; still, slowly I make my progress in this world as I am certain you do as well.

I pray that this letter has reached you with all haste for I have most wonderful news. Since May, I have been traveling through Lower Canada to solicit voyageurs. Outside of Berthier I heard stories of the "man with the hole in his side." Naturally, I made all haste to investigate these rumors & behold I have found him! I have located Alexis.

Ramsay Crooks has long urged us to inform you should we hear of the man. Alas, without your devoted ministrations, he is now poor and miserable beyond description; his wound is worse than when you left it. The hole remains as it was in the beginning.

He is married now and has two (!) children. He ekes out a miserable existence as a kind of day laborer among his kind; I shall not burden you with the sordid details except that he received my visit with his wily kind of courtesy and expressed his Sincere Regret over his flight from your Care and Generous Welfare. He spoke of a Dr. Caldwell from Montreal who has visited him on several occasions. I think he is willing to return to your care and employment should you so desire it.

I could have him sent back to you upon a Company bateau with little inconvenience. I did all I could to bring him up, but could not succeed with these endeavors that cost me $14. I will be obliged if you will let me know whether I should do anything more to get him back and how I shall get my money back as the Company will not allow it to me.

I await your reply and again relay my greetings to you and charming Deborah and darling Sarah.

Your humble servant,
Theodore Mathews
Agent, The American Fur Company

BEAUMONT'S FINGERS TREMBLED. He had to stand up and pace the room. It was as if he had been sleeping for the last three years and now, like some Rip Van Winkle, he had awoken. His once-forgotten investment in the company had reaped its return. He laughed so hard he wiped his eyes. He had actually considered resigning his commission!

He began to imagine the future. Once he had Alexis here he would *have him,* and in time he would have his experiments well done. He would start with measures of temperature and studies of digestion both artificial and natural. Experiments to ascertain the proper temperature of digestion and the effects of climate on it. It was evident the weather was the *primae causa* of ill health and disease and that chemical reactions had a caloric requirement and that digestion was a chemical process. He simply needed to demonstrate how each was connected to the other.

He wanted to tell Deborah straightaway, and he put on his cap and made for the door, but stopped at the threshold. He just let go of the door handle and stepped back into his office, took off his cap and swung it around his outstretched fingers like some toy. He dropped the cap on his desk and sat down heavy in the chair.

"I must be calm, calm but resolute," he said to himself. "And I must be patient. He's found, but he's not yet mine. Caldwell," he murmured. "Caldwell."

He took up the letter again. Dr. Caldwell. It could be a calculated ruse on Alexis's part. It would be like Alexis to do that. Like the drinking trick. Never the mind. Beaumont would marshal the forces of the American Fur Company to take Alexis in hand and bring him to him. Not one cent would pass to Alexis's hand until that hand had grasped Beaumont's.

He composed his reply to Theodore Mathews — *I beseech you, arrange with the Company to have Alexis brought here with all possible haste. Tell him I shall care for the wound as before, and he shall resume his duties as a household servant at a salary of 300 dollars per year.* He included in the letter payment for Mathews's fourteen dollars of expenses. Then he took up another sheet and began a letter to Ramsay Crooks. After some lines about Deborah, Sarah and Lucretia, the death of the infant William, the journey inspecting hospitals and life in Green Bay, he turned to the heart of the matter.

THE ONLY MEN ENTITLED TO HAPPINESS

Remember when we spoke of Science under the canopy of stars on Mackinac Island those many years ago. This is the opportunity for the Company to serve Science and the American People. Alexis is a treasure, and he rightly belongs here in America in the hands of an American doctor. What assistance the Company can offer to assure his speedy travel would be most valuable.

He walked to the clerk's office to post the letters.

Four days passed before he told Deborah about Alexis. It was noon, and they had some two hours alone before they would gather Sarah and Lucretia from the birthday party of Emily, the daughter of Colonel Willoughby, the commander of Fort Howard. They were seated beneath the shade of a maple tree, the remains of a picnic spread before them on an Indian blanket they had bought in Mackinac.

She was stone-faced as he narrated Mathews's letter. When he finished, she smoothed her hands over the flat of her thighs and said plainly, "I had wondered why you were with your notebook."

"My notebook?"

"You've had that out these past days."

She was correct. Since he had received Mathews's letter he had taken his notebook from his trunk and reviewed his notes of the experiments.

"I have been considering whether to complete the treatise on the fevers along the Fox River Valley and considering as well whether it's worth recommencing the experiments with Alexis. It's clear I should, that I must in fact. Science demands it. Progress demands it."

"So then he's to come here?"

"Yes," he nodded smartly. "I've written to Theodore to bring Alexis here. Theodore has been most accommodating; he proposes to secure the necessary resources of the company, a bateau even, to transport him. But when all is done, all is arranged, it won't be any sooner than the coming spring. I'd wish it sooner, but patience is necessary."

"It's strange," she observed, "but I'd not thought of him for several months, and yet for a time he was such a part of our lives. Isn't that funny how we only seem to forget?" She considered her own question. "So then he'll stay here with us as before?"

"Yes. And he'll resume his work as our household servant. I'll let the Hankins boy know he's not needed when the time comes, if in fact we are still here when Alexis joins us. I expect that by next summer we'll be at another posting. I'm long past due for a review of my assignment. Now that I'm a surgeon with eight years service in the remote regions, I've every right to a more settled posting. Soon I'll write to Lovell with this news and a request for assignment to St. Louis."

"Do you think you can secure a post in St. Louis?"

He took up her right hand as if it were some a precious gift and kissed her fingertips.

"I cannot promise St. Louis, but I do have every intention of making that request. We've passed long, long years outside the pale of civilization, endured hardships, and now we've every right to a posting such as St. Louis. I should like to enjoy your singing to the melody you play on a piano in our own parlor."

She tried to smile. "How long, how long do you think your experiments will last?"

"Don't worry, I shall see to it that he has lodging nearby. Not with us. He can do the work as a common household servant and live nearby. I have every intention to foster in him the virtues of industriousness and frugality."

"But how long?"

"Honestly, I can't say. Once, I thought all I should do is prove digestion is a chemical process. But one desire burns in my soul, and that is to observe and to discover, like any good explorer. There is an end to the journey, but I can't claim when it will be. I think that is the fault of many scientists. They claim to know what they want to find, and so they perform their experiments to find just that thing. Their journey becomes almost circular. I shall explore with the singular conviction that this book shall be a book for all to read."

Somewhere a bell sounded the hour. Deborah rose and began to assemble their things. He watched her as she shook out the crumbs and carefully rolled the soiled utensils in a wide napkin.

"Deborah, because this is a medical matter I have not seen the necessity to engage you in its many and multiple details, and yet I know how Alexis is not only my patient but also a household servant. I appeal to you to see that he is an investment for us, much like the investments the company makes. The company's selling ladies' and men's fur hats. That's the fashion now. But Lord rue the day when fashions shifts, as it always does. Think of the man who staked his fortune in powdered wigs. What poorhouse contains him? Alexis offers knowledge of great value to science, to the public. That kind of knowledge is not subject to the whims of fashion."

She stood looking down at her husband.

"What is to say he will not flee again and leave you as bereft as before?"

"Because he comes freely. Why then would he flee if he comes freely and of his own accord?"

"But he was free then too."

"His circumstances have changed now."

"How?"

"He is destitute. Sit down, please."

She remained standing, her hands upon her hips, the blanket draped through the crook of her right arm.

"Don't you see?" she insisted.

"That he is destitute, I'm not surprised. And I'd hazard you're not either. The man tended to intemperance, and judging by the number of children, he clearly has the Negroes' defect in moral and prudential restraint on the sexual connection." He looked at her, and then he looked away. "Excuse me, please. But truly you know the meaning of my words."

"That he is destitute and has a family and has no choice." She entreated her husband. "William, don't you see? He'll stay until he gets what he wants, and flee again, leaving us out whatever dollars you pay him. He does not care about the science of digestion."

She turned away to face the mouth of the Fox River. Two shirtless men were working their way slowly in a rowboat, one at each oar, laughing like boys.

"That's simply part of his calculation, as it is for any man," he observed. "Theodore Mathews wrote that Alexis has worked as a voyageur. I'd venture Alexis must ask himself what this opportunity is worth. There are other doctors. Some Dr. Caldwell has shown interest in him. Alexis has a choice. He could work for Caldwell if he wished. I shall certainly pay him, as I have, and in fact pay him more than I did in Mackinac, for he has a family to support. He comes of his own free will, stays until the work is done, and I, yes I, I will pay him. Man to man. Deborah, could you have the common courtesy to face your husband when he talks to you?"

She did as his courtesy required. "When he left aboard that steamship, you were beside yourself with grief, and now here you are before me wanting him back. I'm just thinking of you and how you suffered when he fled. For weeks you brooded. You mourned. Do you want that to pass again? Do you? What is it you want, William Beaumont? What is it, and will Alexis St. Martin give it to you?"

She folded the blanket and took up her basket. "Come now. We must collect our children."

IN THE DAYS AFTER THE LETTER from Theodore Mathews arrived, ideas for experiments returned like long-dormant dreams. As Beaumont reviewed the contents of his notebook of experiments, plans clarified. He expected he would fill its pages and the pages of perhaps two more before he composed a book suitable for publication on the physiology of gastric digestion, a book that would be read not only by every doctor in the surgeons corps but by all doctors and even the general public. A book that would cross the seas, to London. Even Paris.

That week's work was the usual diseases of warm and damp September days with chilled evenings. Preoccupied as he was with plans for experiments on Alexis, the work he had to do, his duties to his family, Deborah's remarks kindled a panic in him. By Saturday afternoon, his attention flitted over his quarterly report to Surgeon General Lovell, and his eyelids twitched from exhaustion.

It was folly for him to think he had the skill and time to execute experiments. Deborah was right. The man would flee as soon as he got the money he wanted. He began composing a letter to Surgeon General Lovell proposing Alexis be sent to Washington City, where Lovell and his colleagues could perform research, but one Sunday evening, he awoke from a dream.

He was in a theater of sorts, the walls were lined with red silk, and there were men and women dressed as if for a ball. He was looking down on them, from some place between the glowing ceiling and their attentive gaze, and he was talking about his book. He had received some sort of honor, or medal. There were men in robes. People applauded. The room was bright with a kind of yellow light, and bunting hung beneath the boxes. The images grew disconnected. Men were talking about him. His father was among them, bragging about his son, the famous physician.

He lay for several minutes in the darkness, his wife asleep beside him. Deborah was a woman, prone by nature to excessive sentiment, tamed only by Cupid, a quality no doubt exacerbated by her novel reading. It was her nature to let sentiment cloud her reason.

He felt his way in the dark to his worktable and lit a candle, took out his penknife and the notebook in which he had written in the months after Alexis's departure and cut out those pages. He blew on the coals of the kitchen fire, and they glowed and pulsed red like living organs. Then he laid some of these pages gently on the coals, one beside another. The pages smoked, crinkled like autumn leaves and burst into flames. He fed his letter to Lovell into the golden flames. Some pages rose and twisted like feeble ghosts aspiring to haunt other men's dreams, but then they disappeared into ashes and smoke.

NEAR THE MIDDLE OF OCTOBER, a private brought him a letter from Theodore Mathews. Beaumont quickly scanned over the usual pleasantries to find the information he desired.

. . . He says he is eager to return to the service of his doctor and that he regrets his foolish ways of so many years ago, but he has responsibilities to wife and child, and he insists that they should accompany him and that you will employ his wife!!! I tried to convince him that this is an extreme request, that no servant can properly demand, but he insists. She is like him—French Canadian—but speaks not a lick of

English. I suggest that your reply propose to engage St. Martin and his wife to stay with you.

Beaumont stared at the letter. It meant Alexis's two children would come as well. The four of them dependent upon him. He could hear Alexis pleading his case to Mathews. His English would become increasingly incoherent as he became animated with emotion.

"Goddamn and to hell with this!"

"Excuse me, sir?" The clerk on the other side of the room looked up from his paperwork. "Did you ask me something?"

Beaumont glowered at the young man.

"I asked you nothing."

The clerk blinked and swallowed. "Right then." He bowed his head over his paperwork.

Beaumont began to work figures on the back of the letter's envelope. On the one side the expenses of Alexis alone and on the other of Alexis with wife and children. The sums were clear. Pay him less if he is to bring them. They will need just one house. He began to think of things he could not easily express as figures. Alexis having the wife and children, children no more than two years old, would be of advantage to the successful prosecution of the experiments. Alexis would have before him the constant reminder of his obligations as father and husband. As any man, he would have their burden, a burden that cultivated industriousness and made it nearly impossible to slip away in the cover of night.

Beaumont drew a single line though the number 3 and wrote above it a 4. He would pay Alexis 400 dollars per year, and he should bring his wife and children.

{TWENTY-SEVEN}

IT TOOK NINE TEDIOUS MONTHS to arrange affairs. In this time, Beaumont twice considered resigning from the army, but the tallies of his weekly balance sheet restrained him. With the new child and the prospect of studying Alexis, he needed his army commission. It provided a steady income and time both to perform his experiments on Alexis and to cultivate a private practice in St. Louis.

The family would travel south by canoe and flatboat on the Lower Branch of the Fox River. At Fort Winnebago on the shores of Lake Winnebago they'd take the Upper Fox to Portage, where they would cross overland to the Wisconsin River and follow it to the Mississippi River and the trading hub of Prairie du Chien and Fort Crawford. There, they would rest before boarding the steamboat to St. Louis.

In St. Louis, Beaumont was to assume the post as surgeon-in-chief to the Fifth Regiment's headquarters. He had Dr. Lovell's assurance that a private practice was permitted as well. He also had guarantees from Theodore Mathews and Ramsay Crooks that he had only to send word to the company's agents, and they would deliver Alexis and his family via bateau before the winter freeze.

The journey to Prairie du Chien took nearly three weeks. They traveled in a flotilla of two flatboats, each armed with a swivel cannon, and five canoes. Among the passengers was Captain Ethan Allen Hitchcock, whose belongings included a heavy crate marked simply "*Books—property Capt. E. A. Hitchcock*"; Thomas Burnett, a morose Indian agent who read copies of the *North American Review;* and John Marsh, a young land speculator sent by his father from New York who, despite the heat and the dirt, dressed in a silk cravat and vest, kept his mustache combed and lustrous and sat crosslegged on a barrel in the shade of an umbrella. His charge was to secure leases on lead mines in Illinois and Iowa.

The traveling party fell into an easy routine, rising before dawn to breakfast, traveling until a midmorning break for a second meal. Just after noon, they would rest until the shadows lengthened. Captain Hitchcock read Dante, Beaumont reviewed his notebooks, and Deborah took to sketching in her commonplace book. They passed banks lined on either side with golden flowers as far as the eye could see. Once they watched a black bear and her two cubs amble along the banks.

They camped their last night in the shadow of the massive rocks of Grand Gres. The river's steady sough lulled them to silence. Some of the travelers lay back on their elbows and regarded the stars; others gazed into the fire's throbbing glow. The last miles of their trip along the Wisconsin River were swift and easy, and by noon of their last day, the countryside bore evidence they were nearing Prairie du Chien. Captain Hitchcock set aside his Dante to watch the passing scenery, and the young merchant John Marsh nervously asked how much further from Prairie du Chien they reckoned the journey to Monsieur DuBuque's magnificent lead mines might be.

Most of the trees had been cleared, and the stump-stubbled riverbank was increasingly populated with Indian camps. It was midmorning of a hot Tuesday in June when the vista over the bow of the boats gave way to an ever-expanding body of water, and the party first sighted the swirling brown waters of the Mississippi. For Beaumont and his family, this was the edge of the world, Prairie du Chien, the outpost of American civilization.

The northern banks of the terminus of the Wisconsin River were high and flat. The sharp smells of cooking fires and dust and horse urine grew distinct, and wisps of violet smoke hung over the water. They passed the bloated carcass of a pig. The banks gave way to lowlands cluttered with all manner of improvised dwellings and houses. The near banks were soon crowded with people running along the shore, some of them shouting and waving to the boats. The water was teeming with canoes and dugouts and log rafts crowded with men, women and children of all manner of color and dress, calling out greetings and instructions, offering trade and lodging. The air soon grew thick with the dust stirred up by horse and mule and foot, so thick that some bodies appeared as shades and the houses in the middle distance were silhouetted. At the riverbanks, tiny boys stood naked, looking like bronzed cherubs with their pooch-bellied bodies. From somewhere there came the sound of music and women singing. Dogs, some of them as big and dark and long jawed as wolves, barked and ran along the bank.

The young merchant grinned, visibly aroused as he attempted to entice a canoe full of Indian women and girls with what looked like strings of colored glass beads. After a time, he simply laughed and tossed them the beads. Captain Hitchcock was hastily jotting notes in a small notebook. Burnett, the Indian agent, inspected his watch and then the angle of the sun. Now squinting, he consulted his watch again and then sat mutely on a box as the chaos of Prairie du Chien unfolded before them.

"Ain't this place the shit hole of the US of A," announced one of the soldiers sweating at the oars of the longboat.

"Shut yur goddamn foul mouth," the captain ordered from his tiller.

They paddled north up the Mississippi River, keeping out of the river's swift center, past the town of Prairie du Chien on the east and the network of marshes to the west, until they reached an island barren save for the dirty gray walls of Fort Crawford.

They traveled on a canal of slow-running, thick, bronze-colored water that smelled vaguely of rotting vegetables and fish and was crowded with crude canoes, dinghies and dugouts. On the bank opposite the fort, three soldiers stood at the end of a dock that displayed a faded American flag, beneath which flew a weathered regimental flag. Both hung limp and heavy. One of the soldiers whistled and hailed them over, and within fifteen minutes the party had disembarked in Prairie du Chien.

Summer's heat and rains were rotting Prairie du Chien. The marshes smelled of putrefaction, and the populace was overrun by Indians, voyageurs and merchants crowded in lowland heat and dampness. Deborah stood mute as she cradled Lucretia in one arm while holding her umbrella in the other. Sarah clutched her thigh as if it were a tree trunk.

Beaumont shuddered. Prairie du Chien was a place of fevers. They must rest no more than a few days here, avoid the water and proceed with all haste to St. Louis.

At the docks, one of the soldiers signaled to the Beaumonts and pointed them to the base of the bluffs that led to the prairie, to the house of the Very Right Reverend Keyes.

"Yonder by that wooden church. Look for the high fence covered with red trumpet vine," the soldier instructed. "We'll have your baggage sent along straightaway. Go now."

THE REVEREND KEYES'S HOUSE was a substantial whitewashed structure behind a four-foot-high stone wall topped with another four feet of wooden fencing. The aging cleric rose slowly from his chair in the parlor and greeted the Beaumonts warmly. Sweets were brought out for Sarah, milk for Lucretia, and a high-backed copper tub the length of a man was filled. Within the hour Deborah and the children were bathing.

Fifteen years ago, the Presbyterian minister had come west to dispute the Catholic theology and convert the Indian, but he had made little progress with either the residents of Prairie du Chien or the Indians. Within a year, he had lost his young wife to fever. He lived childless, writing his memoirs in his lonely, six-room dwelling.

Beaumont sat with the reverend upon a weathered stone bench in the shade of a great maple in the garden. They were looking out at the overgrown tangle of roses as the reverend explained how rheumatism had crippled him from tending to his garden.

Beaumont surveyed the house and the grounds. "You've a handsome home."

"Thank you. It's far more than I need, fit more for a family such as yours. It's been some years since the charm of a cultured woman graced my hearth. You say you're bound for St. Louis?"

Beaumont nodded. "With all haste. I've much work to do."

"That's a fine city, I hear. Another Boston or Philadelphia. Some say it should be our nation's capital. I grew up in Philadelphia, you know. You're at the edge of it all here on the prairie. When I came here I was all intent to spread the word of the Reformed Church in a free land, throw off the shackles of Catholic superstition and European aristocracy. Convert the Indian. Educate them. I knew not a whit of what precisely I was striding into."

"Progress takes time," Beaumont observed.

"Begging your pardon, Doctor, but this old man knows that time's the problem. History, I mean. The time we know, not the time we hope for. The villagers here claim lineage to traders as ancient as Jean Nicolet in the 1600s. And the Indians, they don't know when they came, and they don't care. We Americans are newcomers. Tyrants, they call us. And I can see their point. After the war, when we took possession of the fort and village, Colonel Chambers ruled with an iron fist.

"There's this story they tell of Charles Menard that's become legend. We found him guilty for selling whiskey to our soldiers, and his house was seized, and he was forced to march through the streets of the village with a bottle dangling by a leather cord around his neck while a band played the 'Rogue's March.' The colonel's punishments soon bore little relation to the nature or severity of the crime. He came to favor banishment in winter on Fever Island, seven miles north of here.

"Now whole families bear grudges, try to claim properties as rightly theirs, produce deeds written in French and signed by noblemen with seals in wax. They'll never forget, and even when they do forget what it is that has them so angered, the memory is like a kind of ancient burl on some great tree trunk, its origins long forgotten. Lightning, wind or ax? Who knows what truly happened? But the mark and anger remain evermore."

The reverend laughed. "The Fourth of July's a spectacle here. The locals take up the 'Rogue's March' as a kind of anthem and carry on with a day's hard labor oblivious to our reverential celebration. Watch yourself. You enter certain taverns, the entire clientele falls silent, musicians set down their instruments, dogs bark like you were some kind of varmint. The innkeep disappears."

"Who has command now?"

"Of the fort? General Zachary Taylor. Nice fellow, about your age. He tries to enforce the laws fairly, but it's a complex arrangement here. The town rightly claims municipal independence from the federal troops. The Indian agents claim the authority of the federal government and its treaties with Indians. But it's commerce that effectively rules us all."

"The company?"

"Aye. Hercules Dousman and Joseph Rolette, the two of them are like brothers, living out of a dilapidated house seized after the war. They've got a steady business selling the Indian agents flour and salted pork, blankets, tools and sundry trinkets to fulfill the treaties, and when we encroach upon more Indian land and violate those delicate treaties, they sell even more to appease the Indians. The Indians become a kind of . . . I don't know what the proper word is, but it's the price of doing business, a kind of debit we cash in from time to time. You say you're going to St. Louis?"

"That's right. I'm posted to the Jefferson Barracks."

"Were it not that my Abigail's buried here, I'd leave this place."

{TWENTY-EIGHT}

IN THE AFTERNOON, BEAUMONT RECEIVED A MESSAGE that Colonel Zachary Taylor wanted to see him. He walked through the narrow red clay streets of Prairie du Chien, stepping carefully past piles of garbage, catfish heads, mounds of ashes, a dead chicken.

On the cluttered dock where the party had landed earlier in the day, a group of seven mud-caked men worked with shovels, boards and mallets to shore up a collapsing bank that threatened to undermine the dock. One of the men looked up and signaled to another who drove his shovel in the muck and climbed onto the dock.

The man was barefoot, and his legs were mud caked to his knees. Only the blue cap pinned with the dull bronze eagle medallion of the First Regiment signified he was a soldier. Beaumont pointed to the fort and explained his order, and the man pointed to one of the canoes pulled up the muddy bank.

"Get in, and I'll paddle ye over."

Beaumont looked at the canoe and again at the soldier. "I can take myself."

"I'll take ye. Need the rest from that muckhole." He motioned with his thumb to his fellow muddied laborers.

As they were crossing the canal Beaumont asked the soldier why there wasn't a bridge to the fort, the space between shore and island being no more than thirty feet.

"Last one plumb washed out in the flood."

FORT CRAWFORD was in rotting disrepair. Years of flooding had turned its lower timbers porous as old sea sponges. In some places, a man could kick the toe of his boot a good inch into the substance of a board, and on many walls the plaster of the first three feet was buckled, water stained and so often patched it resembled an explorer's tentative sketch of a map.

A corporal ushered Dr. Beaumont into Colonel Taylor's dusty office. The colonel gestured Beaumont to a chair and apologized as he scribbled a few words on a document before easing himself back in his chair.

Uniforms among frontier officers were often dingy and worn, but this officer's appearance displayed an almost accomplished disarray. His hair had prematurely whitened and was swept back off his high brow; it had been cut roughly, perhaps by himself without the aid of a glass. His cravat, such as it was, was tied in a loose knot and bore stains, and the uppermost collar button of his blouse was missing. The sleeves of his uniform coat were frayed, and all but one of the brass buttons along the left sleeve were missing.

"I trust the journey was acceptable?"

"Very much so, sir. Captain Derling is an expert river man, and the company was most entertaining. Captain Hitchcock possesses a charming intellect."

"And your accommodations here?"

"Quite fine. Reverend Keyes has graciously hosted us."

"The reverend is one of our most distinguished citizens. He has charge of the school."

Beaumont nodded appreciatively. "The situation was similar in Mackinac. Reverend Keyes's hospitality is superlative."

"I'd like to invite all of you, the reverend and you and Mrs. Beaumont, Captain Hitchcock, Mr. Burnett and the other Indian agents—we've three of them here—my general staff, Misters Dousman and Rolette from the company, to dinner tonight. There are a number of prominent residents at the fort and the town whom I want you to have the pleasure of meeting. Several of the junior officers were at West Point when Captain Hitchcock was its commandant, and Mary, my wife, is most eager to have the pleasure of meeting your wife."

"Thank you, Colonel. We accept your invitation. I know Mrs. Beaumont will enjoy such an evening. As will I."

"The officers here take great pride in our outpost of civilization. Many of them have their wives here. We have assembled a library to rival that of a town back east. Mrs. Beaumont is welcome to peruse it and yourself as well, of course."

"Thank you, Colonel."

Colonel Taylor seemed distracted. He cleared his throat repeatedly. "You've been at Fort Howard. And before that?"

Beaumont narrated his previous postings. At the mention of Captain Pearce, the colonel spoke up.

"It's a tragedy what happened to Captain Pearce. I knew the man from the war. He was with Scott at the invasion of Fort Erie."

"Captain Pearce was a great man and a patriot. I have fond memories of the man."

The colonel nodded.

"It's evident you've experience in these parts, among the voyageurs and Indians. Mackinac and Prairie du Chien are quite similar in that regard, though I should reckon the winters here are far more sociable."

"The Indians were not as visible in Mackinac. They had a kind of village along the beach."

"Your experience is most valuable to the army."

"Thank you, but of course it's all in my duty."

"Certainly. D'you know Dr. Phineas Clark?"

Beaumont shook his head slowly.

"He was our surgeon until near a month ago but had reason to vacate his duty with great haste. I've sent word requesting a replacement. We need at least two physicians here, though we've managed with one. But as the Indians gather to collect their tributes, word spreads of their discontent. The Winnebagos protest that we're taking their lead mines. Clever Black Hawk and his band of Sauk warriors resist vacating to lands west of the Mississippi. Sometimes I think we should have wiped that man out in the last war. But never the mind. The past is past. I've got Indian agents telling me the company's trading liquor to the Indians. The Sioux are furious at the Foxes. Needless to say, affairs are getting complicated. The Great Council of 1825 seems ready to disintegrate, Doctor. I must prepare. We must prepare. Your arrival is most propitious. Most. I expect Indian affairs are soon to boil over. We've been managing with the help of Clark's steward, a young lad named Badger."

The colonel hesitated.

"To be honest, I can't recall the fellow's first name. Everyone calls him Badger. The fellow's good, I'm told, but it's been getting difficult with the fevers coming on as well. A garrison such as this needs at least one physician. Two would be adequate."

Beaumont nodded, uncrossed his arms and tucked his hands beneath his thighs.

"My corporal can show you to the physician's quarters. The hospital adjacent. Floods have been and remain a perennial problem here. You might have noted the waterline along the walls from last year's surge. This was once a modest French structure. When they first settled they should have seen that there wasn't a tree about, but never the mind, London was probably built on a swamp. But this ain't England, I'll grant you that. I've petitioned the secretary of war for funds to construct a new fort on higher ground to the east above the bluffs. When that starts, I'll have men quarrying stone, burning lime and cutting timber. But the space you have is adequate. You simply need to prepare a requisition of supplies, and you have my assurance they'll be sent with all haste up from St. Louis."

"If I may ask, Colonel, when is Dr. Clark to return?"

"Here? I'd expect he's gone."

"And his replacement is due when?"

"Well, that's you until I hear otherwise. I'll send word to the Jefferson Barracks. I've a communiqué to go out within the week."

Beaumont's temples were pounding.

Colonel Taylor rose and stepped around his desk.

"I shall see you at dinner? Seven is when we start with sherry."

He extended his hand. His boots were worn and scuffed at the tips. After they shook hands, the captain kept his grip.

"I, I do know that this is not as you expected. Please understand, I have been posted to over twelve assignments, at least that, and passed some twelve years along this frontier. This is my first posting with my Mary at my side in over two years. I haven't seen my farm in Louisiana in seven years. I had a daughter I never saw. God rest her innocent soul. This is our duty, Doctor."

DEBORAH WEPT. As her husband recounted the meeting in Colonel Taylor's office, she had her handkerchief wrapped around her right hand and was wiping at her eyes. When he reached the end of the story, he embraced her, and she leaned her head on his shoulder, and they sat silently in the lengthening shadows of the afternoon.

They sat on the same stone bench where the Reverend Keyes and Beaumont had sat earlier in the day. Deborah's hair was combed smooth and tied up in a tight French braid, and she wore the pair of river pearl earrings Beaumont had given her upon their marriage. Her robin's egg blue cotton dress, one of her better muslin dresses, fringed with lace, smelled of lavender and cedar. The harshest leg of their journey was over. She had been planning on a few days of rest before their steamboat journey to St. Louis. Beside the swell of her pleated skirts lay her much-worn copy of *Pamela*.

"You could resign from the army."

"I can't do that. You know that."

"You have your promotion," she insisted. "The Griswold affair is behind you and now to be forgotten."

"Deborah, please let's not quarrel over this. We need the steady income the army grants me. I've expended considerable time and money on Alexis. He's an investment that has yet to pay its returns. We need him back."

"Yes, of course," she snapped. She reached for her novel.

By the morning of the following day, Deborah was dressed in one of her gray calico work dresses, sweeping the cobwebs from the rafters and corners of the dusty surgeon's quarters. She beat the spiders to death underfoot.

The place was filthy and cluttered. Only one of the two bedrooms, as well as what passed for a sitting room, bore evidence of human occupation. The other four rooms, including the kitchen, had not been used for months. She quickly abandoned all pretense of dignity. Her dress was sweat stained and damp about her breasts and the crease of her buttocks.

"Did he even eat?" she asked as they sorted through the dented cookware and cleaned out a cast-iron cooking stove in which mice had made a nest.

"Perhaps he took his meals in the mess hall," Beaumont said flatly.

She drew up a list of supplies they required: paint, fabric to drape the windows, new glass to replace several broken panes, varnish for the floor, new mattresses for all the beds. It would take two weeks before the quarters were fit for habitation.

TWENTY-NINE

THE HOSPITAL, LIKE THE NEARBY SURGEON'S QUARTERS, stood outside the fort in a long, pitch-roofed, wooden building. Its weatherworn gray wood was much patched. Beaumont was astounded to find the hospital was over-seen by a boy. The lad was barefoot and dressed in britches that exposed his skinny knees and wore a kind of butcher's smock. His straight brown hair, cut along the rim of a bowl, left his wide ears entirely visible.

"How old are you?"

"About fifteen, sir."

Beaumont simply nodded.

"You the new doctor from Fort Howard?"

"I am. Dr. William Beaumont. And you are?"

"Charles Badger, Doctor. Steward of this here hospital. At your ser-vice, sir." He made a kind of salute with two fingers of his left hand.

"You're Badger. Colonel Taylor mentioned there was a steward."

"That is I, sir."

In an older man, Badger's smile would have been annoying, even mock-ing, but in this short lad, it was entirely endearing. The patients seemed to share an affection for the steward.

"He's Young Badger," said a toothless man who stood with a thin gray towel draped over his head. Several other men laughed and nodded. The man then hobbled to his narrow cot. One of his legs was bandaged and ev-idently lame.

Beaumont looked about the room. It was perhaps double the size of the hospital at the Mackinac garrison, more akin to one of the hospitals in Plattsburgh during the war, with tandem rows of twenty cots each along a long corridor. Windows were spaced at regular intervals, except many of them were covered with boards. The light that filtered through the dust and grime of the remaining panes caused those panes to glow. The cots were evidently not sufficient as there were blanket rolls set between some of the beds.

In August 1828, two months after Beaumont arrived in Prairie du Chien, he managed a note to Theodore Mathews: *We are not settled in St. Louis. Duty has assigned me to Fort Crawford for an indefinite tenure. I will send news whether this shall change, but until I receive further orders, we remain here, and Alexis should come here upon my word.*

There were rains, and the multiplying chorus of frogs sang a kind of nighttime prelude to the fevers to come. After the rains, as the heat grew steady and withering, the stagnant pools in the flooded marshes turned green and began to bubble. The fevers came. At first, the cases were sporadic, but in time, they multiplied: an entire platoon of soldiers on hay-gathering duty, whole households, developed bone-shattering agues, some so violent they squeezed the very marrow from their bones until they pissed black water, while others suffered mild shivers that only interrupted dinner conversation. Badger and he made an efficient team. The lad was skilled at the lancet and sorting the treatable sick from the few hopeless cases.

Beaumont ordered Deborah and the children to keep away from the village, to rest in the shade of a dry place, to wear shoes and drink only the water from the springhouse. During the worst of the fevers, he was away from home for days at a time, sending messages that he was well and receiving notes in her elegant cursive that they too were well. The ladies had organized a reading salon, and little Sarah was learning needlepoint.

The French villagers soon came calling for the doctor's help. By autumn he had collected or was owed a handsome tally of fees from the merchants and traders and tavern keepers. The fevers abated, but there was no pause in Beaumont and Badger's labors. Construction of the new fort on the plateau above the town had begun. Crews were detailed to gather lumber, there being not a usable tree within six miles of the fort, to cook lime and to haul stones. Those assigned to clear the land on the plateau found centuries' worth of bones, skulls and vertebrae, smooth clay pots with images of running animals, jagged lines and whorls, obsidian tools whose fine edges looked to be worked with tiny hammers. They carried these relics out in barrows and tossed them over a cliff into the river below. The pots exploded on the rocks.

Injuries multiplied, a fractured jaw, smashed hands, cuts deep to bone, and in winter, frostbite and delirium. Work on the new fort continued until the winter storms came, whereupon the soldiers retired to the fort and rested until the spring thaw. Some of the soldiers made a hobby of fashioning toys or scrimshaw with the Indian bones. The officers put on the English comedy *Who Wants a Guinea?* They transformed a barracks into a theater; painted scenery hung from canvas drapes. Bayonets with candles secured into their grips served as improvised lighting. There were three tiers of seating: the first for officers and distinguished citizens, the second for soldiers and white laborers, and the third for the Gumbos, Negroes and Indians.

In February of the New Year, just before Lent, the French villagers of

Prairie du Chien spent many evenings in the taverns and grog shops, lit lanterns and torches to illuminate the dirty snow-packed streets and roasted whole goats and sheep upon spigots. They drained kegs and smashed the empties to add to the bonfires. They danced in a frenzy until dawn. Then on Ash Wednesday they stood patiently in line before the priest, as he recited a Latin phrase and used his thumb to smear ash on their foreheads. In the forty days following, they composed themselves in a sullen display of tipsy penance. On Easter Sunday, they dressed in their finery, slaughtered lambs, lit fires and drank and danced again.

By winter's end the Winnebago had accepted a treaty that reinforced their claim to the mines and guaranteed twenty thousand dollars compensation for the trespasses upon their land in exchange that no harm would come to white men who trespassed. The United States would pay the Winnebago for the damage done by the white man. Though disagreements existed with the Chippewa over lumber they claimed had been unlawfully taken from their land, Agent Burnett was confident that with enough presents for the tribe he could broker an arrangement.

But the spring thaw seemed to unleash dormant passions, both Indian and white. Borders were once again in dispute. Allied bands of Sauk and Foxes were furious at the Menominee and Sioux for transgressions upon their land. Chief Blackhawk was once again agitating that his former land in Illinois had been unjustly seized, that the treaty of 1804 which set in motion the subsequent treaties was itself null and void. He promised that he would cross the Mississippi to make corn on the eastern shore, on the land he claimed was rightfully his tribe's.

Captain Hitchcock had news from Washington. He had returned from hurried travels up and down the Mississippi River to forts Snelling, Armstrong and Edwards to coordinate the army's response to the Indian agitation. The recently inaugurated Jackson administration was sending more Indian commissioners west to reopen negotiations with all the tribes, but the captain was privy to Secretary of War Eaton's secret orders. Erase the Winnebago, Pottawattamie, Ottawa and Chippewa Indians' claims to any land east of the Mississippi and south of the Wisconsin River. Drive the Indian west.

Hitchcock and Beaumont were returning from a morning bird hunt in the plains above the village near the site of the new fort. The incomplete structure glowed white in the morning sun. They walked with their fouling pieces over their shoulders. Captain Brown's speckled bird dog trotted in a zig-zag before them, its pink nose on the ground before it. Each man carried a brace of pheasants that turned on their leather cords. Their knee-high boots were slick with dew. Hitchcock was bothered by all that he had seen and heard.

"This notion that Burnett and the rest of the agents have that the Mississippi River is to be the boundary of our progress — I consider it a fiction. Have you seen the steam engines that race along two parallel iron rails? What shall stop one of those from traversing this river on a bridge like the London Bridge? A mere river is not going to stop our nation's ambition. We will drive the Indian to the very shores of the Pacific."

"I understand those engines are delicate contraptions."

"You've seen the Erie Canal, have you not?"

"Aye. I've one of the medals that commemorate the construction."

"Well then? There you have it. A canal of water. Rails of iron."

The two men walked on for several minutes.

"I fear," said Hitchcock, "that further covenants, agreements and treaties with the Indian are simply a means to an end, not to be valued and upheld. It's war by another means."

Beaumont considered the point.

"We might be here for years then."

Hitchcock nodded slowly.

THAT EVENING AFTER DINNER Beaumont explained the situation to Deborah.

"What does it mean for us?" she asked.

"It means that this is not a temporary stay. By June, July at the latest, this place will be overflowing with Indians of all tribes. Hundreds, perhaps thousands will gather for a council. By all events, we shall be here for some time, and it shall be busy."

She continued scrubbing a pot.

"I am certain I could arrange for you and the children to go on to St. Louis."

"Don't be silly. We are a family."

He watched her as she worked over the dishes.

"I'm not going to let this stop me, you know. I shall write soon to Theodore Mathews to have Alexis sent down. Pierre Reynard has agreed to lend out a set of rooms for Alexis and his family. It will not cost a cent. It's in return for the care I gave to him and his family."

Deborah did not pause in her labors. "Family?"

"Pierre has a wife and five children. I cared for them when they had the fever."

"You said Alexis's family."

"His wife and children. He insists on coming with them. I told you."

She wrung out her dishrag and draped it neatly over the dowel. "You did. Yes, you did. You will be busy. We will be busy."

"Please, Deborah, don't be sharp like that."

"I'm not being sharp, just stating a plain fact. What will she do?"

"His wife?"

"Yes, of course."

Beaumont shrugged. "Take care of his children, I should expect. She's not our charge, that's for certain. Neither she nor those children. He's a man now. If there is one virtue he shall learn it is industriousness. As I see it, having his family here will keep him settled. They'll remind him of his responsibilities. It will make him a better man. And it will keep him here."

He thumped the tabletop with his forefinger.

She stood before his chair as he looked up at her. "It will be odd having him back after all that happened, has happened."

He reached up and took her hands.

"I'm sorry, Deborah, that things have not worked out as we planned. But with him here I can resume the experiments, and in time, please don't ask me how much, I'll have that book done, and with that we shall have our fortune, and I can resign this army or, better yet, have the pick of the best assignments. And the world will be a better place for our sacrifice. My book shall change the world."

"I know that, William. I do. I just want us to be happy. To be happy in the pursuit of happiness, if such a thing is possible, that is my prayer for us."

"Events are out of my control."

"You know what I think."

"Resign? Debbie, I can't simply quit."

"But you have your promotion. Your reputation redeemed. We've spent more than five years beyond the pale of civilization. Surely, William, you could set up a private practice in St. Louis? The city is booming. You yourself have said that a private practice there will be lucrative. It's likely to be the new American capital. So why then must we suffer here? They could just as well send us back to Mackinac. You plainly disdain the military authority on your practice. It's Alexis, isn't it?"

"What're you saying?"

"As long as you have your post, you can take the time to study him."

"When the book is published, we can leave. Until that time, I ask for your patience."

"It has been more than five years."

"That is entirely enough, woman! Private practice? An apprentice-trained physician from Vermont? I suppose I could succeed. There are all kinds of snake oil vendors up and down the Mississippi." He waved his arms to demonstrate the vast scope of this commerce. "Even Dr. Ben Franklin worked and sacrificed before wealth was his and as he wished. Unless you have some greater plan to secure our wealth and station, I should think you should see the wisdom of patience. That is *my* prayer."

Deborah stood red faced before her husband, then turned to her washbasin.

IN APRIL, Beaumont called upon Hercules Douseman and Joseph Rolette at their cluttered house inside the American Fur Company compound. The traders were preparing for the season of commerce with the Indians. The warehouse was stacked high and tight with goods; more goods overflowed into their house. The dogs snaked between the boxes as Douseman led Beaumont into the room he and Joseph used as a kind of kitchen and sitting room. The place smelled of fried meat and coffee.

Beaumont produced a letter.

"I was wondering if I might ask a favor of the company. I'll pay, of course. This is for Theodore Mathews. He's one of your agents."

Douseman nodded. "Little Teddy. Up in Lower Canada."

"Yes, him. I could send it in the U.S. mails, but I was wondering if you can see that it gets sent with the next bateaux convoy you send up the Fox-Wisconsin waterway?"

Douseman took the letter, inspected each side and slipped it into a pocket within his leather vest. He patted the spot.

"We've a boat going out within the week for Green Bay. He'll have it within four weeks. You'll get your answer by June."

"Thank you so much, Hercules. How much do I owe you?" Beaumont reached into his coat pocket.

"Nothing, Doctor. Put your purse away. Courtesy of the company. I know that Misters Mathews and Crooks want to see your Frenchman back with you. That fellow with the lid over his stomach. St. something."

Joseph Rolette was nodding. "Martin," he announced. "Alexis St. Martin."

Beaumont looked from Rolette to Douseman. He stammered.

"I didn't know."

"You got friends in good places," Rolette said. "We'll see that you get your man. There's not a brigade in the entire Upper Mississippi that will hire him. He's as good as yours. Your man." He dropped his jaw and let out a great guffaw of laughter.

❦[THIRTY]❧

AROUND NOON ON THE 29TH OF JUNE, 1829, a clerk from the American Fur Company interrupted Beaumont at his work bandaging a soldier's leg wound.

"Mr. Douseman sends me to tell you, Doctor, that the reply to your letter has arrived."

"Well then, hand it over."

Beaumont held out his right hand. He snapped his fingers.

"At your house, sir. Mr. Douseman says they're there waiting for you."

Beaumont lowered his hand.

"They are here?" but he did not hear the sullen clerk's reply. "Badger," he called. The lad turned from his work rolling bandages.

"Sir?"

"Can you finish with this dressing here? I'll be back by the by, or to-morrow."

Beaumont had risen and was making to wash his hands in the basin. The soldier with the wounded leg lay propped up on his elbows. He looked at the clerk. The clerk shrugged his narrow shoulders. Then the soldier looked to Badger.

"Tomorrow, sir, is Sunday, sir," said Badger.

"It is. I'll see you Monday then. You have the day as we discussed."

"Yes sir. Thank you, sir."

ALEXIS WAS RECOGNIZABLE even from behind, even with his straight black hair tied into a ponytail. He had the same broad shoulders and long arms and slender waist.

He must have seen Deborah's relieved smile when she spied her husband, for he turned to see his doctor striding toward them. Deborah, Sarah and Lucretia, Alexis and beside him a short woman in a kind of loose-fitting, knee-length dress tied up with a length of cord around her waist. The ends of the cord were braided and beaded and knotted to keep from fraying. She was holding a moon-faced infant in her left arm and waving her right hand to shield it from the sun and keep the flies from its face. A small boy clung to her skirts.

As Beaumont approached them he felt his pulse quicken and his face warm. He was thinking that at least one year had passed since he had done any reading of substance on the physiology of gastric digestion, and there was much reading still to do.

"*Mon Docteur Beaumont.*"

Had he grown? Perhaps an inch or two. He seemed more a man now.

"Alexis. Alexis St. Martin."

They grasped hands.

"Welcome to Prairie du Chien."

"Thank you, Doctor."

They still shook hands.

"Alexis. This is a surprise. We did not know you were to arrive. It was only this past April when I wrote Mr. Mathews. We thought we'd be in . . ." he hesitated. "But never mind. Now here you are. Here."

Alexis nodded, grinned.

"I am. Thank you, Doctor. Thank you. I am at your services."

Beaumont finally released his grip and looked to Deborah. He wiped his brow with his sleeve.

"When did they arrive?"

She smiled at Alexis as she spoke.

"Just a few minutes ago they came up with one of Mr. Douseman's clerks. The boy from New Orleans."

A wheelbarrow stood nearby, piled high with two trunks and several canvas-wrapped bundles tied with the same cord that Marie wore as a belt. Alexis nodded vigorously and pointed to the barrow.

"We've just had the chance to talk before you came. Let me introduce you to Marie St. Martin," Deborah continued.

The small woman who stood behind Alexis blushed at the sound of her name.

Beaumont looked at the child clinging to her legs. The barefoot boy could not have been more than five years old and was dressed in a kind of smock that reached below his knees. The garment was filthy. The child's face was tanned and his eyes nearly obscured beneath his straight bangs. Flies swirled about him. They swirled about everyone.

Alexis held out his arm in a gesture of presentation.

"Dr. Beaumont, my savior, I would like to make a present to you of my Marie. Marie, this is Dr. Beaumont." Then he chattered quickly and quietly to her in French.

She stepped forward tentatively.

"She speak no English," Alexis announced, his own accented English drawing out the *i* like a long sharp *e*.

Beaumont took her small hand. Her face was round and pox marked, and she wore her hair parted down the middle and pulled back into a kind of bun, though several strands hung free and were stuck with sweat to her temples and cheeks. She could not be more than twenty years old.

"Hello, Marie. Welcome to Prairie du Chien. Welcome. I am Dr. Beaumont, and you have met my wife, Deborah, and my children, Sarah and Lucretia."

He pointed to each as he pronounced their names.

Marie looked at him with large brown eyes.

"*Allo, Docteur Beaumont*," she whispered and managed a kind of curtsy.

Alexis leaned down to the boy who still clung to his wife's skirts.

"And this is Alexis, my son. He is four years old."

He held up four fingers to more clearly demonstrate the child's age.

"And this is Charles. Born just this past fall." He stroked the infant's cheek as he gazed at him. "He traveled well."

Marie turned to her husband and chattered in rapid French. Her husband replied forcefully, but she cut him off, gesturing with her chin to the infant Charles. Alexis ignored her and turned to Deborah.

"Where is little William?"

Deborah cleared her throat. "The child is not with us anymore," she said.

Beaumont stepped close to Alexis and put his hand upon his bony shoulder. It felt as thin as it had some five years ago.

"This child died. In the winter four years ago."

Alexis frowned. "I am so, so . . ."

It was Deborah who spoke up.

"Alexis, Marie needs some milk for Charles, no? Milk? *Du lait*? The children look hot and tired. Let's get them something to eat and drink. Come." She signaled that everyone should follow her into the house.

IT WAS EARLY EVENING when Beaumont returned home from the hospital. Around sunset, a great wind swept in, and the massive clouds that had gathered in the east blew in over the prairie, and within minutes great drops began to slap the hard-packed road. Soon a wall of rain poured down. Beaumont would have lingered in the hospital until it passed, such showers always did, and he had much work still to do, but it was long past his supper. He was hungry and lonely for his family. He picked up a square of planking from the side of the road and held it above his head. The villagers ran to gather up laundry and other implements. A band of some fifteen Winnebago braves, well covered under animal hides they draped over their heads and shoulders, watched them. They were part of some five hundred who had come up from Rock Island for the great council.

As these braves passed, some of them eyeing him coldly and steadily, he recited to himself a line from a poem the salon had read in Fort

Howard. *'Tis war alone that gluts the Indian's mind, as eating meat inflames the tiger kind.* The articles and covenants and treaties and presents were ceremonies of war. He missed Mackinac Island for its order, the separation of the Indians from the white men and its isolation from the Western frontier's passions. It was good that he had allowed Alexis to bring his family here. They would keep him settled and contain his wild and uncultivated habits.

He stood in the doorway of his house, dripping from the waist down. Deborah and Sarah came laughing to his aid. They helped him pull off his muddied boots and rain-soaked trousers. Deborah wiped one boot clean while Sarah held the other boot, intently watching her mother. They set the boots and clothes to dry before the stove, and Sarah sang a song about the rain.

When he returned from the bedroom wearing dry clothes, Deborah had already taken out his plate from the warmer and placed it at his place at the table. She, Sarah and Lucretia were seated nearby on the floor, their dresses spread out like flowers in full bloom. The girls were playing with dolls. Deborah was working on her needlepoint. He sat, lifted his brocaded napkin from the plate and took up his fork and knife. After a time, he set down his fork and watched his wife and daughters.

"Rain was so bad it fairly poured into the hospital. I need to tell Colonel Taylor to dispense with the repairs to the roof. They ought to simply tear that thing down and build a new one. Makes no sense to use lumber on that roof what with how scarce lumber is. I can wait a few more months."

Deborah nodded. "Marie was here after you left."

"When? This afternoon?"

Deborah nodded.

"And?"

"She needed more milk for the children and brought some kind of bread she wanted to bake in our oven."

"And a mop and a bucket." Sarah told her parents that Mrs. Martin wanted to clean her house.

Deborah blushed. "I lent her a mop as well. That old one that was here when we arrived. And one of our buckets. The leaky one. I'll fetch them back on Monday."

Beaumont looked over at the oven.

"But she doesn't speak a word of English."

"She carried an empty pitcher and a bowl full of dough, and her gestures are fairly demonstrative. She's not as shy as she seems, you know."

He nodded.

Deborah guided Sarah over to the washbasin in the children's bedroom. She returned cradling Lucretia and stood before her husband.

"I know you'll get the mop and bucket back," he said to her. "You know, on the walk over to the Reynards' she was chattering like a jaybird to Alexis. The Indians seem to have her worked up. I don't think she's seen them before, at least not in these numbers and these wilder kind. There's a whole band of Chippewas come up from Rock Island, and that's not even the half of them. I'll speak with Alexis about the milk and the stove. Their rooms have a kitchen that's theirs to use as they wish. I showed it to them when I dropped them off. It's a perfectly acceptable stove, and they can buy or trade for milk just like the rest of us. He was a lad in Mackinac, but he's a grown man now, and it's his duty to learn to be independent of our charity. Man to man is how it shall be between us. He gets a salary."

"How is he?"

"He looks thinner, but he's clearly in reasonable constitution. That journey was what, some two thousand miles, and they made it in three weeks. Of course, most of it's over water, and those bateaux move quickly. He said he helped with the rowing, said it reminded him of his days as a voyageur."

He pushed his plate away. "I'm sorry about his remark about Little William."

"How could he have known? I meant how is his side? You know." She held her right hand over the place on her own body.

"I haven't had occasion to examine him yet. As soon as I dropped them off at the Reynards' I had to return to the hospital." He exhaled heavily and began rubbing his eyes. "The Second Regiment is due soon, and I want to have things in order. I've so many cases now I simply can't keep track of them, and Badger asked for tomorrow off, so I've got to go in tomorrow as well. These rains and crowds of Indians and soldiers mean the fevers will surely come, and Burnett is hounding me to talk to Colonel Taylor about prohibiting the sale of whiskey to the Indians. Can you believe that? Might as well order the rain not to fall. Douseman and Rolette want the man run out, but it turns out Burnett knows President Jackson. The two of them rode circuit together in Tennessee. Imagine that, Burnett knew Andrew Jackson. It promises to be a busy, busy summer.

"But don't worry, if the hole isn't there or Alexis isn't amenable to proper experiments, I'll pack them all up in the next bateau and have them shipped back to Lower Canada."

THE ROOMS AT PIERRE REYNARD'S were set in an outer building built in the last century. Its mud bricks were melting, and several stones had spalled and burst from their mortar. The living space consisted of one stone-floored room with a sand-floored kitchen space in one corner, and one other low-ceilinged room that served as a bedroom. There was a table, several chairs and crates, and along the walls shelving and mounted peg boards. The windows, all four of them, were covered with oiled cloth. The doorway into the large room was wide and closed by a double door that swung upon great iron hinges. The air smelled of horses. The stones in the northeast corner floor were darkened with dampness.

By Saturday evening, after a meal of beans, bread and catfish and with the children put to bed, Marie St. Martin had drawn up a list of the items they required to make the space habitable.

She stood before Alexis enumerating these items as he sat staring into the small fire that burned in their rusted stove. He dangled a flyswatter made from a length of dowel and a square of found matting. He had given up the hunt. The black specks crisscrossed among the crumbs on the table-top. She wanted a proper door for the stove, a pot that could fit snug into the cooking hole, new sand for the kitchen space, screens for the windows to keep the flies out, fresh straw for the mattresses, a proper latch for the outhouse door, a broom, a bucket that did not leak like the bad one the doctor's wife had lent them.

"That's enough," he snapped.

"I have one more hand to go." She held up her hand and balled her fingers into a fist.

"I said that's enough, woman. I'll talk to Dr. Beaumont."

The baby began to cry.

"When?" she insisted.

"As soon as I can. We just arrived."

He slapped the flyswatter on the tabletop and leaned forward with his elbows upon his knees. "Goddamn, this chair hurts my ass. Aren't you tired from the journey?"

"I'm exhausted," she said. Then she burst into tears.

THIRTY-ONE

THE TWO MEN WERE SEATED, FACING EACH OTHER, Beaumont on a milking stool, Alexis on the edge of a cot. A low table stood beside them. The oil lantern glowed and winked. Beaumont had set these furnishings up in a corner of the barn adjacent to his house. It seemed the proper place to inspect the wound and to conduct experiments. It was close enough to Beaumont's house to permit Alexis to easily interrupt his chores, but also separate from both house and hospital, where Beaumont was certain one and twenty distractions would divert him from his work with Alexis. In the summer, the space was cool as the barn was among the oldest buildings in Prairie du Chien, with two-foot-thick walls constructed from flat stones. In the winter, a stove kept it passably warm.

It was just after dawn, four days after Alexis and his family had arrived.

"Now then, why don't we have a look? Your shirt."

Alexis pulled off his shirt, tossed it in a heap on the cot and sat with his hands gripping the edge of the cot, his elbows flexed outward.

"Sit up a bit, please."

Beaumont directed the lantern light to better illuminate Alexis's chest.

A saucer-sized area of flesh below his left breast was dark, thick and twisted with scar tissue. It undulated with the tempos of Alexis's heartbeat and his breathing. At its center was a pucker of pink tissue, like tiny lips signaling for a kiss. The unmistakable surface of the outer coating of the stomach gathered into the valve.

"You don't dress it?"

Alexis shook his head. "I thought today not to do so as we would be together."

"But usually?"

"I wrap a cloth about it."

"Does it bother you?"

"Bother?"

"Hurt?"

Alexis looked down at the wound.

"No, Doctor. Not at all. No pain. My wife, she says it is ugly. I have to wear a shirt when we are together."

"Well, that's not unusual. I'm sure she doesn't understand it as we do. Lie back on the cot, please."

Beaumont tapped the surface of the thin mattress.

"Mr. Mathews mentioned a Dr. Caldwell. In Montreal or thereabouts. Did he do anything with the wound?"

Alexis became demonstrative with his hands as he lay on the cot. "No sir," he said. "I would not let the man touch it. No man has touched this except you. You are the one I trust. I promise to God that only my savior Dr. William Beaumont can touch this."

Beaumont nodded. "Right then. Just keep your arms at your side. Let's have a closer look." He scooted the stool closer to the edge of the cot.

It was just as he had last seen it five years ago. He put his left hand on Alexis's side; the diameter of the hole fit like a coin between the tips of his outstretched thumb and forefinger. Alexis flinched.

"Does that hurt?"

"No sir." He giggled. "Just tickled a bit."

Beaumont moved his thumb and forefinger. The lips slightly opened as if to speak. There was at least some give in the tissues. He put the tip of the index finger of his right hand on the pink tissue. He pressed gently. The tissue was soft, smooth and warm. His finger easily passed to the first knuckle.

Alexis made a kind of grunt.

Beaumont kept the finger in place. "What's that?"

"That, that sense."

"The tender cuticle of the edge," Beaumont explained. "It will pass." He continued to advance his finger until its entire length was inserted into the warm and moist cavity of Alexis St. Martin's stomach.

"How are you?"

"*Bien.*" Alexis said softly. His left forearm was crossed over his face so as to cover his eyes, and his head was slightly turned to the wall.

"*Bien,*" Beaumont repeated.

When he drew the finger out, the valve was only partly closed. He directed the lamplight closer to the cavity. The pink and folded tissue of the inner lining of the stomach was visible. It was glistening, and it was beautiful.

He set the lamp back. "The wound looks good."

"Thank you, Doctor."

"Cough please."

"*Comment?*"

"Never the mind."

The release of the valve had allowed the gastric tissue to flower through the hole. The tissue blossomed until it presented itself like some shining, rugated, pink rose. Beaumont gazed at this for several minutes. He ran the pad of his index finger over the warm, slick surface and touched that to the tip of his tongue. The taste was slightly acrid. Then he applied three fingers to the center of the bloom and gently eased the tissue back into its hole. This done, he pushed his stool away from the edge of the cot.

"Up, up," he commanded.

Alexis swung his legs over the edge of the coat. The pink tissue of the valve fell into place and entirely covered the hole. Beaumont gazed at the wound for several moments. When he spoke he had to clear his throat; his voice sounded low and hoarse.

"There it is as it was. Well then, why don't you put your shirt on? I want to show you our garden plot, and we can take some tools there. It's in dire need to weeding and such, and I've got some netting that needs to cover the lettuce."

Alexis finished tucking his shirt into his trousers. He pushed his hair behind his ears. "What about this?"

"About what?"

He pointed to his left side.

"Not today. I have to be at the hospital. Tomorrow, meet me here in the morning before your breakfast. And here." He reached over to the peg where he hung his coat and took from the pocket a folded piece of paper. "This is half your first month's payment. I thought it sensible to grant this to you now so you can get settled. Buy things you need for the house and such."

Alexis snatched the paper and opened it. He counted the bills.

"Doctor, if you please, I would like the rest of the month's pay?"

"The rest?"

"For as you say the costs of things here. My wife, she has a long list."

Beaumont pointed to the cash Alexis had stuffed into the pocket of his trousers. "Why don't you see how that does you, and we can discuss that later? You need to learn to exercise frugality. And I nearly forgot, when Mrs. St. Martin's done with her cleaning, please return the mop and bucket she borrowed."

"It leaks. The bucket leaks."

AFTER THE FIRST EXAMINATION, Beaumont managed a few quick observations of Alexis, no more than measurements of the temperature and the flow of the clear liquor from the empty cavity. But these efforts were hasty. He had no time to dedicate to his research. All the tribes were now assembled at Prairie du Chien.

The agents had doled out some twenty thousand dollars to the Indians in goods—barrels of flour, pork, corn, pipes and tobacco—and cash with promises for at least another fifteen thousand dollars of the same. The place was now a seething mass of sun-baked men and animals. The Indians greeted the arrival of steamboats full of goods with fusillades of rifle and musket shot.

In time, the idle braves grew bored and insisted their daily allotment of the meat of two oxen be delivered alive. They took these massive beasts to the prairie and set them loose under the pursuit of riders mounted bare-backed on ponies and horses, some of the mounts painted like their riders.

Armed with spears, bows and arrows, they pursued the oxen across the prairie, at times in a running line, then fanned out, then back in line, one hundred braves, pursuing the oxen until one of the beasts stumbled forward, flipped on its snout and lay heaving upon its side, a bleeding mass of prickled arrows and spears. Its companion turned and lowered onto its forelegs as if to make a stand. The Beaumonts and the St. Martins were among the crowd of cheering soldiers and residents of Prairie du Chien who witnessed the warriors circling their quarry. A Sauk chief dismounted and with a war club in hand, walked smartly up to the heaving creature and smote it upon the crown so that the head exploded in a spew of blood. Then the creature came down in one exhausted, blood- and mud-covered heap. Colonel Taylor banned the sport.

Beaumont's work at the hospital doubled and doubled again. He and Young Badger set up a second hospital tent. The sight of an idle Alexis was like beholding an incomplete chore brought to life. He was determined not to see his funds wasted and assigned Alexis more and more chores at the Beaumont house and garden plot. He ordered him to weed and trim plants, cut irrigation ditches and carry water up from the river by donkey to fill the barrels, cover the corn with netting to keep away the birds, plant a crop of winter potatoes. He brusquely criticized the work even as he assigned him more.

Alexis grew despondent, his clay-dusted face streaked with sweat and tears of anger. Many evenings, he shuffled home from the grog shop numb with drink. Marie waited for him with her arms crossed upon her stout chest, her hair matted with sweat. Regardless of the heat, she kept the house closed up, the great doorway latched, a musket at the ready. The Indians terrified her. By the last week of July, they had run out of the money Beaumont had advanced them and were living on vegetables from the garden, catfish and the charity of Pierre Reynard's daughter for milk.

Marie shuddered. "We traveled all this way, all of us, so you could be a peasant farmer?" Her dark eyes were wide with anger. "We gave up all chance of settling in Berthier, an entire growing season, and here we are now doing exactly what you could have done at our home, among our family, our people, who care about us, instead of here among strangers, savages and a landlord who treats us as common servants. You working side by side with Negroes. Me begging for milk, playing the meek one to coax the doctor's cold wife for laundry soap."

"That is enough! Enough!"

"It is not enough," her voice was lowered but sharp. "I smell your breath. You drink away all our money. You promised me that there would be money to have here. Easy, quick money and no labor other than a few chores. And that we would be gone before the freeze, and what do you tell me? That we are here for the season to harvest his potatoes? And he has not once done any of his tricks with your stomach? Why are you not then a voyageur? If you wish to travel, leave us in Berthier where we are safe, not here among the copper-colored niggers!"

He stared at his wife for some time. He shuddered as he exhaled.

"Because I can't find a job as a voyageur. No one will take me on. You know that. They found me. They know my name. They know who I am. The moment that Mathews man found me, they never stopped calling. It's like they are searching for me. You would think that in all of Canada, the Northern territories, a man could strike out and get away from his past and his name, but I cannot. I can wear a shirt, but even then I cannot hide this."

He gestured to his side.

"Even if I lie about who I am, they will see this asshole in my side, and then it's done. The doctor has some great power. I swear to you, Marie, the hand of God works through him. He can find me and draw me here. But once we're here, I cannot control the things he does to my stomach."

"When will he be done?"

"He hasn't even started."

"Why?"

"I do not know, Marie! He's been working. Some days he does not even speak to me. I come here, and he is as my best friend, draws off a few vials of the water, and now he can scarcely tolerate my presence."

"So then we harvest potatoes and hide in this house from the Indians? Come winter we freeze and beg for food because you drank it all."

"Marie, you know I don't want to be a farmer. It ruined my father in body and soul. I am a voyageur. A proud Blackfeather, but if I cannot do that, then I shall do what I can to make good money for my family. Eight hundred livres is some good money. It's my hope, my prayer, that Dr. Beaumont gets what he wants from the wound, finishes his tricks, and we get our money. Then it is all done, my debt is paid, and I can return as a voyageur and shall never have to see him again. This will not go on forever. I will be free of him."

She stared at him. He was gazing at the floor. He was weeping.

"And I hope too, some days, that he might heal me."

Marie sneered and waved her hand as if to swat at a fly.

"He saved my life, Marie. The man is brilliant. God worked though him. I cannot just spurn him."

"And God has left him. A fallen angel."

THE AUGUST SUN WAS RELENTLESS, drying out the ponds and swamps and turning the fields brown and dusty. By noon, the smell of rotting fish and vegetable matter was so intense that even the dogs avoided the marshes. In the evenings, the fires were lit, and the sounds of singing, drums and pipes would last long into the night. The Indian agents' insistence on a strict policy of no whiskey sales to the Indians only raised the price on a barrel, so that within weeks some tribes had exhausted their presents and were begging for corn.

Beaumont began to quarrel with the St. Martins over items borrowed and not returned, the cause of a broken bowl, the damage to a carving knife blade. Alexis demanded his salary paid early. Beaumont refused it. He forbade Lucretia and Sarah from speaking French. One Saturday morning, he ordered Marie St. Martin to cease her chatter and slammed his door on her reddened, tear-stained face.

Distant prairie fires burned. In the evenings their glow was visible from the hills above the village, and the haze of smoke obscured the sun until it became a pale yellow disk that no more burned a man's eye than a guttering candle. Bits of ash fell like negatives of snowflakes.

In the middle of August, the great council began. The army set up a large canopy beside the fort, and Beaumont joined the officers and Indian agents arrayed in their finest dress uniforms. The collection of white men and Indian dressed, ornamented and painted was like some burlesque show of Babylonian dimensions. They were a display of gold braids, crimson fringes, plumed caps, brass and polished black leather. The officers and soldiers joked that old rough-and-ready Taylor was now fancy, dandy and diplomatic. The Indian chiefs dressed in robes of ermine or buffalo. They braided beads and feathers into their hair, or tied their hair up in a kind of pompadour and struck it through with porcupine quills. Silver armlets circled their great biceps, and their spears and bows and ax handles were ornamented with shells and feathers and colored ribbon. Some had their faces painted white or red, and others displayed handprints on their backs and chests.

{THIRTY-TWO}

AT THE END OF SUMMER, A MAN APPEARED at the hospital dressed in the uniform of the surgeons corps. His trousers and jacket were unusually clean and well fitted, and he kept his mustaches in the great flowing style that was the fashion among St. Louis gentlemen. He carried a black leather doctor's bag with the initials *J.D.E.* embossed in gold beneath its handles. Behind him was a Negro who pushed a dogcart piled with trunks and cases. He stood at the doorway and inspected the hospital structure. Beaumont stepped forward to greet the man.

"I'm William Beaumont, surgeon of the garrison."

"Dr. John Emerson, Third Regiment."

The two doctors shook hands.

"Welcome to Fort Crawford. We've been waiting for some time for you."

Beaumont followed Emerson's gaze to the rafters and the patchwork of ceiling repairs. "I don't deny it's a shabby space. Colonel Taylor promises a new structure."

Emerson nodded. "They sent me directly here, but I don't hazard this is where you live?"

"No, this is the hospital. This and the tent out back for the overflow. My wife and children and I live yonder in that house. We long ran out of beds once the fevers began. Rains started a week ago. Like clockwork in the afternoon."

Emerson held his hand to shade his eyes as he looked back at the whitewashed fort, glowing in the morning sun. "You think they'd put me up in the fort? Seems the best place with all these savages about."

"There's quarters there."

Emerson called over his shoulder. "Dred, this here is Dr. William Beaumont."

The man nodded and smiled.

"Dr. Beaumont, this is Dred Scott. He's a good and loyal boy, and I've taught him some of the skills of a surgeon's mate. Dred, why don't you wheel our belongings to the fort, and don't leave them until I return in a few hours. Dr. Beaumont and I have some work here."

"Yes sir." The man began to move away with the cart.

"Dred," he called. "You got some change for a meal?"

"I do, sir."

"Right then, off with you."

Emerson turned and stepped past Beaumont into the hospital.

"Well then, Doctor, let's get to work. Hotter than Hades here, and more flies swirling than round a latrine. Here then." He had unbuttoned his uniform coat and handed it to Badger. "What's your name, boy?"

"Badger, sir."

THE GREAT COUNCIL carried on for some two weeks, and in that time the doctors worked day and night, some days tending to as many as six new cases of swamp fever and an assortment of injuries. With the end of the council in August, their work began to lessen enough that Emerson was able to enjoy a day of bird hunting upon the prairie. One afternoon, the doctors sat in the shade of the hospital, drinking tea and eating cold beef sandwiches. Emerson sat with the back of his chair tilted against the side of the hospital, his long legs stretched out and crossed at the boots.

"Why do you bother with that Frenchman of yours? I see how you get frustrated with him. The man's near useless. You ought to get yourself a proper Negro like Dred."

Beaumont stared at the riverbank, where several herons made slow progress among the reeds.

"How long have you had Dred?"

"I've owned him outright now for two years. Got the title in my bag. Bought him off a family in St. Louis. Fellow named Peter Blow, a Virginian come to St. Louis a few years back, died, and then his children sold off the lot of slaves. Dred's traveled with me through the free state of Illinois and the Iowa territory for at least a year now. Fact, I left him in Rock Island for a spell when I had to make it back quick to Jefferson Barracks. And not once did he make a petition for his freedom or so much as take a step to flee. You know why?"

Beaumont shook his head slowly.

Emerson was enjoying his disquisition.

"He's on his own with charge of my luggage. He could run away with a handsome set of belongings. But he won't, and he won't petition for his freedom. That's because I'm good and loyal to him, and I take care of him. I trust him like my son. Ours is a relationship of mutual benefit. I'm not like one of those plantation owners I expect you've read about in the abolitionist pamphlets. You know Taylor's got a plantation?"

"The colonel?"

"That's right. Colonel Zachary Taylor has himself a handsome plantation in Louisiana with some two score or more slaves."

Beaumont considered the point. "I'm sure he's a kind master."

"He may be. But what of his overseer? So, you didn't answer my question. Why do you bother with that Alexis fellow? He's as lazy as an Indian and clever as a fox. All those Gumbos are. And never mind that wife of his."

"I don't disagree with you about her."

"Well?" Emerson insisted.

"It's complicated with Alexis. Many years ago, he was a patient of mine. I expended a considerable effort to heal his wound, a gunshot blast to the lower chest. He owes me a considerable sum for some three years of support I provided as he healed."

"Never paid his fee then?"

Beaumont nodded. "In a manner of speaking, that's right."

"I suppose that's a fair arrangement between men. A kind of an indenture, though I've come to see those as problematical agreements. Owners tend to work the fellow to death seeing as the time is limited. Mind you, William, I ain't implying you're doing that. It's just a general observation. He doesn't seem very good at what he does. I just do not see why you put up with him."

"The wound he sustained healed in a most interesting manner." Beaumont began to explain the wound and the plans for experiments and the book. When he finished, Emerson whistled.

"Now I can see why you're hangin' on to him. You might make a handsome profit with a book like that. People love to chatter about their bowels and their various pains and hypochondriacal lamentations. It's a pity he's not a Negro 'cause when you own the man outright, it's a kind of investment you got to protect and nurture, and he just follows the orders. That's in their simple nature. 'Course you can't own him. He may be a Gumbo, but he ain't Negro." Emerson snapped his finger and laughed. "Say then, why not get him enlisted in the army? Treat him like a soldier. Hell, he drinks like one. Dred saw him at the grog shop the other week put away some seven whiskeys, and then he stood up from the table with barely a sway to his step. I'd a been on the floor. Flat out like a board."

Beaumont laughed.

"What's wrong?" Emerson asked. "You never seen him do that?"

"Oh, I have. I have heard of it. But that's not the cause of my laughter. I'm the cause. Me. Several times I've thought of resigning the army. My wife pleads with me to do so, but you've given me the idea I've needed. This plan of employing him as a servant is nonsense. He doesn't want to be a servant. More to the point, he can't be a servant. And I actually had this sentimental notion that having his family here with him would kindle his sense of responsibility. That is as much a folly as what the Indian agents like Burnett dream for the Indian. He's a wildflower. It's simply not in his nature to be an industrious citizen. The trick will be to get him away from his family. Far away and in uniform."

BY SEPTEMBER, the Indians had departed. The daily affairs at Fort Crawford and Prairie du Chien soon settled into their usual routines. The foundation and walls of the new fort on the highlands overlooking the village were completed. The roof would wait until the spring. Colonel Taylor ordered the work crews to cease construction and focus on laying in firewood for the winter. The commodity was growing increasingly scarce, with work crews needing to travel as far as ten miles to locate adequate timbers. The garrison of soldiers was reduced by half. Dr. Emerson was among those transferred to Fort Snelling. On the day Emerson departed, Beaumont embraced him and thanked him.

THIRTY-THREE

BEAUMONT WAS INSPIRED WITH THE IDEA of enlisting Alexis and moving with him to a posting where Beaumont would have only light military duties, if any at all, away from their families, where he would have complete control over Alexis. He would sketch out the considerations and negotiations necessary for such a posting along the frontier, in St. Louis, or back east, but none of his ideas could fulfill all his desires and plans. He felt the frustration of his years when he was a schoolteacher and he was struggling to advance to a greater profession. Each day, he grew more despondent.

By November, he was quarreling with Deborah about Alexis. Alexis's work was shoddy, he was often drunk, and Beaumont had not yet done a single experiment. When Beaumont discovered that Deborah had given Marie two of her old dresses, he flew into a rage.

"They're short on money," she explained.

"You haven't given her money as well, have you?" he snapped.

"Of course not, William. They're just old dresses. Juliet Roulette says they fight constantly."

He stared at his wife.

"Do not look at me like that. I gave her some old clothes that I haven't worn in years. Dresses that don't fit me proper."

It was late in the evening, and they were seated at their kitchen table.

"I don't doubt Alexis has run though his money. The man spends and drinks like an Indian. But that is no reason we should turn him and his family into our charity cases as well. You see how the Indians just take and take. There's no bottom to their desire. It's a game for them. That's just how Alexis and his kind are."

"William, they were my clothes that don't fit me."

"I paid for those clothes. We can get fair value for them. The company buys such things."

"To sell to the Indians."

"To sell to whoever buys them. Who cares? We could use them for rags as well."

"William, we've plenty of rags. Plenty. I'm not going to quarrel with you over the value of some old dresses that do not fit me."

Beaumont slapped the tabletop.

"I should never have consented to him bringing his family along! The man's an ungrateful patient and a clever manipulator. They play at poverty, mind you. *Play* at it. God only knows what money he's got stuffed in a shoe somewhere, and yet his children walk about barefoot and in rags. I get so frustrated with him needling me for money, complaining that garden tools break, doing nothing to solve a problem but only presenting it to me like some lazy steward during the war. They are like Indians. Worse even. You mustn't encourage this behavior."

Deborah gasped. "William Beaumont, what has possessed you? You are the one who said that the man is an investment. Should those dresses manage to placate Marie, all the better, what with the quarrels you've had with her. You wanted them all here, and now you have them. And if he's an Indian, well then, why don't you shoot him if he disobeys his treaty!"

They stared at each other. She was red faced. His nostrils flared. He made to speak, a kind of low noise from deep in his throat, but instead he stood and walked out of the room.

BY DECEMBER, the winter sun hung low and dull in the Northern sky, and the days stayed well below freezing. Wolves were about. Prairie du Chien was winter locked. Six months had passed since Alexis had arrived, and Beaumont had not managed one experiment. He feared that to start the experiments would only anger Marie and provoke Alexis to leave. To take such a chance was foolish. But he could not think of a plan to take Alexis away from his family, and yet he was still paying the man. Finally, after a week of sleepless nights, he decided to start with experiments that required little of Alexis's time.

He drew a firm line in his notebook and wrote beneath that line, *To Ascertain the Relative Difference between Natural and Artificial Digestion.* Just after seven on a Saturday morning, Alexis St. Martin lay on his back on the cot in the barn with his green flannel shirt unbuttoned and pulled open to expose the aperture to his gastric cavity. In addition to the lamp, Beaumont had set out in a neat row several clear glass vials and their corks and his gum elastic tube.

"Nothing to eat yet?"

"No, Doctor. Nothing." He held his right hand over his heart.

"Good then. I'll have a look in a bit." He fussed with the vials and the tubing.

"You recall the gum elastic tube? I used it before to gather the juice."

Alexis nodded.

"This will only take a few minutes, and then you can get to your breakfast and back to your chores. You hungry?"

Alexis nodded.

"Good then." He reached for the tube and eased its tip and the tip of his forefinger against the pink tissue at the perforation. It slid in easily.

Alexis winced.

"The tender cuticle," Beaumont announced.

Beaumont slid the tube as far as it could pass, and then he drew it slightly back. He kept the ball of his right thumb sealed over the end of the tube. In his left hand he held one of the empty vials.

"Now then," he said, "onto your left side."

He held the vial under the end of the tube and removed his right thumb from the end. Nothing came. He jiggled the tube. Nothing. He passed it in and out with short strokes. Several clear drops passed into the vial, then a few more. After five minutes, Alexis moaned. Beaumont had gathered only a drachm or two.

"That sinking feeling?"

Alexis swallowed hard. He nodded.

"Well, that's it." Beaumont corked the vial, slid the tube out and lay tube and vial neatly on the tabletop. "Why don't you fix yourself up and get to breakfast?"

Alexis lay for a moment with his eyes still closed. "You're done?"

"Yes."

Alexis sat up. "Is it all well? I felt like I was falling and sick."

"Everything is fine. That's just the effect of the gathering of the juice. You've had it before. Can I see you back tomorrow morning, before your breakfast, please? That will be Sunday, so then it's not a problem as you fast before the church."

After Alexis left, Beaumont stared at the meager sample of gastric juice he had gathered. It was not sufficient to study artificial digestion. It would take several days to gather more. For the next four days, Beaumont simply measured the temperature of the cavity when Alexis was fasting. These measurements took all of six or eight minutes, and as he kept the tube entirely still, they caused Alexis no distress.

The data on the temperature were interesting, but of greater value was the effect these simple measurements had on Alexis. He was now comfortable with the simple penetration of the cavity. Seven days after the first effort with the elastic tube, he set to work upon Alexis. After considerable irritation of the cavity with the tube, he gathered just two or three drachms, but by Monday evening he had managed to gather one and one-half ounces. He now possessed nearly a vial full of the juice. That afternoon, he added twelve drachms of recently salted and boiled beef to the vial of gastric juice, and he recommenced his sand bath experiments.

For twenty-four hours he tended to his sand bath, keeping it as close to blood heat as possible and gently agitating the vial. After the first six hours, the solvent action seemed to cease upon the beef, and it was nearly half dissolved. He used his scalpel to dissect the piece with as much precision as possible to separate the undigested from the chymous portions. Then he squeezed the chymous portion through a thin muslin cloth until it was dry. He weighed it. Five drachms, two scruples and eight grains. He worked the simple math out in his notebook. Some six drachms and twelve grains of the beef had been digested. A ratio of two to one. For every drachm of aliment, some two drachms of gastric juice are needed.

He wrote furiously of the implications of this ratio. A meal of too great a weight would overwhelm the production of gastric juice and consequently, as evidenced by the beef in the vial, produce the symptoms of indigestion. That failure of the system could lead to putrefaction of the aliment. Natural digestion was chemical. Putrefaction and fermentation were pathological.

There is always disturbance of the stomach when more food has been received than there is gastric juice to act upon it.

In the following weeks, he sampled meals and mixed the samplings with ox gall and bile. In March, Alexis began to protest the experiments. One morning, after Beaumont had drawn off a vial of gastric juice, Alexis sprang from the cot and assumed a defiant posture. Beaumont sat passively in his chair, his face cast in stone, as Alexis ranted that Beaumont had not an idea of what he was doing and the irritation it caused: the sinking feeling when he stuck the rubber tube inside, the pain along the edge.

"Just poking about like some, some, I don't even know the word for such a perverse man!" he screamed. "Marie is right. I should double my fee for this. Double it!"

Alexis turned on his heels. Beaumont followed him to the doorway. He called after him. "I'll deduct that fee from the two years of charity you owe me. And your life." As he watched Alexis stride away, he spoke to himself. "You're a fool, William Beaumont. An utter fool. Bringing this man and his family into your care. Your own personal Indian tribe." He spat. "Emerson was right. Undo this mess and get him alone and reserved in a barrack somewhere. But where? How?"

⟨THIRTY-FOUR⟩

IN THE MIDDLE OF MAY, JUST AFTER SUNRISE, a soldier summoned Beaumont and his family to hurry to the fort with all possible haste. Within the hour, the streets of Prairie du Chien rang with whoops and shouts and wicked laughter and screams. Some two hundred Menominee and Sioux warriors came streaming through the streets and alleyways, twisting and dancing and leaping.

They were dressed for war in leggings or colored breachclouts, their bodies painted red and black, and they carried their slaughter. The heads of Sauk and Fox men and even some women were stuck on poles that they swung and pumped up and down, turned to and fro, so that the one faced another and then another in rapid succession, as if talking like puppets in a macabre theater, their bloodied locks of hair slapping each other. Men wearing necklaces made from ears shook spears decorated with coal black scalps. Some of the braves kicked a head back and forth like a ball.

The American soldiers lined the fort with rifles ready and pitch pots smoking beside the swivel cannons. The Indians outnumbered them three to one. In time, the Indians moved off to a field, and there they kindled a fire. Rumor spread that they roasted and ate the heart of the murdered Fox chief. They departed before nightfall.

That evening, when Beaumont returned to the room where Deborah and the children were kept, he found her sobbing. Her sewing was a confused bundle on the tabletop. The pepperbox pistol he had left for her sat beside it.

"We must leave this place," she begged him. Her face was swollen, her eyes red. "We must."

He held her close. He stroked her head.

"We will," he murmured. "I promise you. I'll figure out a way."

BY JUNE, reports of Indian hostilities and threats upon the settlers came regularly. The Indians argued that the treaty of 1804, the first treaty and the foundation of subsequent agreements and treaties, was coerced from them, unjust, and thus all subsequent treaties were null and void. The settlers and farmers along the Illinois River demanded the governor call out the militia. Sauk Indians inspired by Blackhawk were tearing down their fences, stealing livestock and potatoes, claiming the Americans stole their land. Similar stories came from the lead mines in Iowa. Troops were dispatched throughout the region, and the garrison at Fort Crawford doubled its size. Colonel Taylor ordered the work crews on extra shifts. He wanted the new fort completed by July.

The heat became oppressive, swarms of blackflies swept in like thunderclouds, and the place was soon covered in a fine red dust stirred up by the horses and wagons, the soldiers and merchants and officials with the Indian agency. For much of June, Beaumont accompanied a party of soldiers sent on a mission north in pursuit of a rumored war party of Sioux braves. Young Badger was left in charge of the hospital. The terrain soon became sufficiently difficult that they abandoned the supply wagon, divided up the goods and carried them by pack. They scuttled their ten-pounder cannon, stuffing its barrel with dirt and rocks, smashing the wheels and pounding lead into its firehole. They tossed the shot into a pond.

They rode through fields thick with weeds that reached to their horses' necks, traversed swamps with mud holes that sucked a man to his waist. Snakes fell from trees. In the evenings, they wrapped their heads in cloth and tried to sleep as they coughed the smoke of green-wood fires, anything to drive away the blood-hungry mosquitoes.

After two weeks marching, Beaumont's guts ached. His bowels ran. There were rumors of cholera in the territories. He dosed himself with laudanum and counted his years, backward to his birth in Lebanon, Connecticut. Forty-five. Too many with too little accomplished. One night, he used a finger length of wood from the fire as a carbon and scratched in his notebook, *I am running out of time.* After four weeks of wandering, the captain in charge ordered the mission aborted. It was mid-July when they returned to Prairie du Chien, their mounts blown, their uniforms shredded, much of the powder they carried turned to clay.

AT THE END OF JULY, one afternoon, Beaumont paused his work organizing the hospital records of the last several months. His desk had papers scattered across it. Badger was an able hand at physic and surgery but inept with records.

Beaumont reached for a rag to wipe his forehead. He wiped his arms as well to keep their dampness from smearing the ink on the pages before him. His shirtsleeves were rolled high above his elbows. He was fanning himself with a folded pamphlet one of the newly arrived officers had pressed upon him. It presented an illustrated attack on President Jackson and his administration, complete with cartoons of Indians suckling on the Treasury Pap and the Little Magician Martin Van Buren directing President Jackson with a wand.

He had been thinking about the results from that winter's experiments. The rule describing the ratio of the gastric juice to aliment seemed less logical. It would surely vary as a consequence of the purity of the aliment, and the admixture of aliment and juice would vary as well with other secretions, other articles of aliment. In the weeks since Alexis stormed out of the barn in a rage and before the Indian hostilities began, he had managed only few short experiments.

"You fool," he said to himself. "You ambitious fool. You should just sail away from here."

He needed time. Time he did not have. And he needed control over Alexis. He tossed the pen. Its ink stained the curled paper.

He looked up. He gasped. Alexis was standing at the threshhold of the open door.

"Alexis, how long have you been there? Dammit, what's the matter?"

Alexis surveyed the crowded desk.

"I remember your office in Mackinac. It had those things on it. The green stones you said came from a man's insides."

"Much of those things are still packed away since the move. I've substantial paperwork to tend to now. What is it?"

"Marie—my wife—she, wants to leave. My wife wants us to go back to Canada."

Beaumont nodded. He gestured politely to the chair.

"Sit down, Alexis. Please. Just put those things on the floor." Beaumont motioned to the only chair beside his in the office. It was stacked with papers and ledgers.

Alexis set them on the floor, and the stack toppled and spread out like a line of waxed playing cards spilled from its pack.

"*Oh, mon dieu.* I am so sorry." He began to gather them back into a stack.

"Never the mind about that, Alexis. Just leave them be."

Alexis looked up at the doctor.

"Just leave them there. There. Leave them. Now sit. Sit, please. What's this about leaving? When?"

"As soon as we can."

"You can't be serious. Why?"

"The Indians, Doctor. She is terrified."

"So is Madame Beaumont. We're all terrified. But Prairie du Chien is secure."

"Doctor, she is not happy. Since we arrived, she has not been happy. I try, but she is too sick for home. She wants me to go back to farming. She says this is no place to raise a family. I beg your leave."

Beaumont exhaled through his nose.

THE ONLY MEN ENTITLED TO HAPPINESS

"She's right of course," he said plainly. "She should go. This frontier is not a proper place for civilized women and children such as ours. Perhaps in another decade it shall be, but not now. But I wouldn't leave now, not now with the Indians as warlike as they are. There is no telling who they will attack next. Or where. But I have a plan. I have a plan for us to leave." Beaumont took in a great breath as he regarded Alexis. His heart was thumping into his throat. "Alexis," he asked, "have you ever heard of Paris?"

"Paris?"

"Yes. The capital of France. Of all of Europe. Where Bonaparte ruled."

Alexis nodded.

"I propose we go there. It shall be better travels than those as a voyageur. And more lucrative and certainly better work than work as a farmer."

"Which is what I do now."

"Alexis, those won't be your chores once we are on a great ship across the ocean. You won't have any chores. And you shall be paid. Paid a good wage."

"Away?"

"Paris is where medical science reigns supreme."

Beaumont had no idea where this inspiration came from, but he liked it as he listened to it. He stood up and dragged his chair around the desk and set it before Alexis.

"Alexis, listen to me. I know you are frustrated. So am I. This is no place for our work. No place for our wives and children. But we must be patient. You leave now, and you will very well find you and your wife and children taken hostage into an Indian camp. I've been in the wilderness, and I have felt the fear. You take your family back to Canada now, you put them at grave risk. But when it is safe to travel, I can easily arrange it with the company, at no expense, in a convoy. I will follow with my family to settle them in Plattsburgh, New York, with my cousin Samuel. When I arrive there, I'll send word through the company. Join me there, and we will depart for Paris."

"But my wife, she would protest this."

"Protest the money and her being among her kin?"

"Protest my absence."

"Just as you would be if you were a voyageur, which is what you want to be, right, not some farmer?"

Alexis regarded his doctor for several moments.

"I could bring them."

"No. No, I don't think you will. You know you don't want her along. One year in Paris, Alexis. You will never, in all your life, have such a chance as this. You will see palaces where kings have lived, where Bonaparte was crowned emperor. Father Didier once lived there, you know. Do you remember him?"

Alexis nodded.

Beaumont smiled. "He told me of his years there at the monastery. You could visit there too."

"And what if I choose to stay in Canada?"

"You'll be a farmer," Beaumont pronounced.

"I can work as a voyageur."

Beaumont looked into the teepee of his hands pressed palm to palm as if in prayer. Then he looked at Alexis. He still looked like a boy, his face oddly unblemished and smooth, but he was not a boy anymore.

"Don't be silly, Alexis. Heavens, but sometimes I feel I'm not just your doctor but your father too. The only men entitled to happiness are those who are useful. I pay better money than the company, and they won't hire you. You know that. Not the Hudson Bay people either. It's a big territory, but it is a small world. Look, Alexis, I don't want to argue with you. I propose this one year, you and I together, good wages for you, all expenses paid, and then it is done."

Alexis looked over at the dirty window. Several blackflies, some near the size of coins, walked along the pane as others futilely flew against it. The small thud of their flight halted by the wall of glass. The corpses of a few lay along the gray sill.

"Sometimes," he said, "I wish I had let you sew it up. Sometimes too I wish that my prayer was not answered, that I had just died."

"Alexis."

Alexis looked back at Beaumont.

"You know that Negro man Dred? The one who served the doctor with the fancy clothes?"

Beaumont nodded.

"He called me a white nigger."

Beaumont sneered, waved one hand before his face as if to rid the air of a stench.

"Alexis, you're a free man. I bought your indenture so I could destroy the document. I pay you good wages. And better wages soon. Dred's a slave. Three-fifths a man. Besides, think of all that I did for you. On the day of your shooting, they wanted you to be in the storeroom. But I resisted them. They wanted you cast off in a boat when your wound still spilled food like a spigot and you were scarcely able to hold a hatchet. But again, I came to your aid. I always have, and I always will. First and foremost, you're my patient."

Alexis laughed. "You have me there. And here too. You are very clever, *mon Docteur Beaumont*. And I am your servant."

The two men looked at each other for some time.

"When might we leave?" Alexis asked.

"I have to make arrangements. I shall speak with Misters Dousman and Rolette. In time, you and I shall be sailing to Paris."

After Alexis left, for several minutes Beaumont remained in his seat, staring at the chair where Alexis had sat. He rubbed his face. This plan was intemperate, to be sure, but it felt right and proper, like the morning when he tossed his pen down and ordered Elias Farnham to come with him to the company store and fetch the wounded trapper.

THIRTY-FIVE

THREE DAYS LATER, HE TOLD DEBORAH HIS PLANS. It was a Sunday, after church and before supper at the Taylors'. The morning was clear and cool. They were walking through a mown field, their daughters running ahead. Deborah held her Bible up to her chest, the strip of red felt ribbon lapped over the leather cover. Her face was shaded by a wide straw bonnet. When Beaumont finished talking, Deborah continued walking. After a minute, she spoke.

"I said I would follow you anywhere, even here, but why must it be Paris?"

"Considering the expenses, it would just be Alexis and me. But Paris is just an idea, Deborah, a plan really, to allow you and the children to get away from here and back to civilization. The surgeons corps is short of doctors. Given my lack of seniority, I've little chance of persuading them that I deserve a posting back east, but I do have Alexis. If I can persuade Dr. Lovell of the value of devoting myself to studying Alexis instead of trying to fit that work together with my regular duties, I'll complete the book. First, I need to secure our leave so that we can return to Plattsburgh, and you and the children can settle there. I'm certain my cousin Samuel would take us in. For at least a year."

"Why not perform your studies in Plattsburgh?"

"He'll be less than two days' journey from his family there. He'll simply take the money and flee north."

Deborah shuddered. She made to speak, then caught herself.

"What is it, dear? You don't want me to go, I know."

"You think you will be done with him after a year?"

"Done?"

"With the experiments."

"I would expect yes, if I can diligently apply myself without the interruption of practice and the duties of a garrison. I need Alexis alone and without the distractions of his family. That wife of his is . . ."

Deborah interrupted him. "You know she's pregnant."

"He's not said a word. How did you know?"

"You can't tell? Look at her face, her chest. All the signs are there."

"Honestly, I've not paid notice. The woman avoids me."

They walked for several minutes.

"So much the better then," Beaumont announced.

"What's that?"

"That he is to be a father again. Now he'll have four mouths to feed. An infant shall require him to remain here until at least next spring and further obligate him to his family. He doesn't want to be a farmer. He can't be a voyageur. What skills does he have? His only thing of value is his wound. If virtue and wisdom do not let him see the debt of gratitude he owes me, then let the duties of family and fatherhood compel him."

"Do you like Alexis?"

Deborah had stopped walking and raised her head so that the shadow of her hat lifted from her face.

"Like him?"

"Yes, like him."

He stammered. "Honestly, Deborah, I often wish that someone such as Captain Hitchcock had suffered that wound. He'd be right here by my side, intent on discovering the secrets that will improve the lot of man. Eager to repay his debt for my efforts. To do something of value."

"Would he have a debt?"

"What do you mean?"

"I'm not sure, really. Would a man such as Captain Hitchcock have required our charity in Mackinac?"

"Deborah, I haven't the slightest idea. Perhaps not."

"The captain is our friend, William."

"And perhaps, too, he is wise enough to see the value of being studied by the greatest medical minds rather than dithering with some country doctor in a barn on the edge of civilization."

She said nothing but looked at their daughters.

"I'm on the edge of greatness, Debbie. I think how far I have come since I was a mere surgeon's mate during the war, often ignored and expected to stand against the wall while the doctors gathered about the table to discuss cases. If I can persuade Lovell to grant me this leave, I shall be seated at that table among the leaders of the surgeons corps. I had occasion several nights ago to review the notes I took from those first four experiments. I've managed considerable progress, despite my amateur skills. The wealth of knowledge that wound has to offer is tremendous. And it is mine."

"It is. I know that," she said. "And I know Lovell supports you, since you were in the army, like you were his son."

She stopped talking.

"Why do you chuckle?" she asked.

"We are of the same age."

"Lovell?"

"Aye. In fact, I'm older by three years. And yet when we met in the surgeons corps in the war he was my commander. Surgeon-in-chief, graduate of Harvard College with a doctorate in medicine, and I a mere surgeon's mate. Apprentice trained. You're right, of course. It's just queer, given our ages."

"Well then, I'd surmise he's like a brother to you. Look at all that he's done for you. As you say, and have said before, we have come this far; just a little farther, and we will have made our fortune. But Paris?"

"Debbie, a man such as Lovell is born into the world with all kinds of advantages, but a man such as I has to make his way by dint of hard work and diligence and daily application of body and soul. I wish that I had the opportunities of a man such as Lovell, but I was not so fortunate to be born of a fine Boston family. I must go away to do this work. Think of this as war, Debbie. I was called away for one month in the futile pursuit of those Sioux, and I very well may be called away again. These experiments I have done and still need to do upon Alexis are of the same kind of duty; I am just as bound to see their success as I am to serve in a war. This research is like war. But there is one difference. Just one. Do you know what that is?"

"No, William, I don't."

"I'm the commander, the one who will have just and fair claim to the fruits of our sacrifice, and I intend to use every possible means to see to their success. Lovell likes me. That is why I remain in the army. I have his support, and I shall use it to its fullest to finish this book. Were I simply in private practice, I'd not have such a powerful friend."

"You say it shall be for just one year?"

He nodded.

She shuddered.

"Hold me please, William."

He wrapped her in his arms. The sharp edge of her Bible cut into his chest.

"I love you, Debbie."

"I love you too, William."

15 September 1830
Dear Dr. Lovell,

The situation being as it has been on this far western frontier, I fear my letter of the 1st of August has not yet reached you, or if it has, that your reply is entangled in the confused transport of materials & supplies. And so forgive me, but I am compelled to write again for I remain anxious to obtain a period of leave from my garrison duties for one year in order to devote myself fully and tirelessly to experiments and observations among the medical

THE ONLY MEN ENTITLED TO HAPPINESS

185

experts of the East Coast as well as those in Europe. My Frenchman is eager
to make this trip & see these places. I am certain he shall come.

I implore you sir, to see to the Justice of my request. With an election
year looming in Congress I fear that our Legislators will have little concern
or inclination to help in the affairs of the medical department. Hence, your
urgent action is needed. I have been banished from society and compelled to
live outside the pale of civilization for 14 successive years constantly at
arduous duties. Privation, hardship and injustice are imposed on a few
medical officers long stationed on the extreme frontier. Officers of every other
section and department of the service are freely and frequently granted
indulgences. The officers of the northwestern frontier should occasionally get
the same.

Despite the conditions of the place, the considerable hardships my family
has suffered, I have dedicated myself tirelessly to creating one of the finest
Hospital establishments in the army. Should a replacement surgeon not be
readily at hand, I recommend without hesitation my steward, C. H. Badger,
a most able and proficient physician and fully competent to assume the role as
physician in chief in the interim. I would feel confident to entrust the medical
duties of the command to this young man than to employing any physician in
the vicinity of Prairie du Chien for their lot are itinerant, speculating
Doctors in whose talents, or integrity I could neither repose confidence, nor
even recommend to the employment of the government, with half the
cheerfulness & safety as I could Young Badger.

For personal reasons relating to his wife and family, Alexis must depart
soon for Canada & I out of duty have granted him this leave but I fear that
with every month away, his duty to me will Evaporate & that once He is in
Canada, the English doctors will lay claim to Him and he will be lost from
us forever.

> *Sincerely,*
> *William Beaumont, MD*
> *Surgeon, U.S. Army*

Beaumont became the model of efficiency and military precision. In September, when the inspector came to survey the hospital, he kept the man busy for two days listening to detailed discourses about the proper instruments necessary for a modern garrison hospital and the need for a replacement set of surgical tools. He proposed a list of books that should be mandatory at all garrisons, urged the purchase of a barometer and thermometer.

In the months before Alexis gathered his wife and three children to depart Prairie du Chien, as the spring melt set in and trading routes began to reopen, panic rose in Beaumont that his plan would fail, that Alexis would never rejoin him. The panic drove him to work. He studied Alexis daily, collecting vials of gastric juice, setting up his sand bath and measuring the pace of digestion there and in the cavity of Alexis's stomach, sampling the contents hourly: venison steak, the white of two eggs, roast beef, roasted pig, wild goose. Every supper for weeks at a time.

Each event displayed new facts. The effect of two days of fever showed masticated food insoluble in Alexis's stomach. Beaumont concluded the importance of withholding food from the stomach in febrile complaints. *It can afford no nourishment; but is actually a source of irritation to that organ, and, consequently, to the whole system.* Early one afternoon, while Beaumont sampled the chyme from a breakfast of pork, bread and potatoes, Alexis rose up from his cot and snapped *"Ça suffit."* He began yelling in French.

"Easy there, Alexis. Speak English."

Alexis just stood there, red faced, the angles of his jaw pulsing.

"Is there some problem? Some pain?" Beaumont gestured to the stomach. "You've nearly digested," he insisted.

Alexis only shook his head slowly.

"Well then, would you please lie back down?"

Within a few minutes, Beaumont observed how yellow bile now tinged the chyme. It was glorious work, making sense of the common wisdom of medicine that anger retarded appetite and produced a bitter bile in one's throat. Conclusions were irresistible.

On April 12, 1831, one year and ten months since Alexis arrived in Prairie du Chien and three days after Alexis's last supper under Beaumont's hourly observations, Beaumont met the St. Martin family at the docks of Prairie du Chien.

A work crew was busy tearing out the dock's rotting planking as Alexis loaded his family's belongings into a company bateau. He was careful with their bundles and trunks, taking care that they were snug and well packed. He helped his wife step into her seat; then his son handed his mother the infant Henriette.

Beaumont extended his right hand.

"Farewell, Alexis," he said. "You needn't worry about writing. The company shall keep me posted. I'll call on you as soon as we arrive in Plattsburgh."

Alexis shook Beaumont's hand, then stepped into the boat.

The St. Martins were bound for the Ohio River via the Mississippi. As Beaumont watched the line of four boats dipping their oars to make their way downstream into the middle waters of the Mississippi, he decided one year would not be adequate. In these last two months he had discovered wonderful things, and there was so much more to discover. He wished to repeat an experiment he'd done a few weeks earlier in which he'd compared digestion of a parcel of food suspended in the stomach, to another in the sand bath, to a third vial tucked under Alexis's arm. The idea of axillary placement of a vial had come to him late one evening in an inspiration. He saw this as a method to reproduce the natural variations in the body's temperature without the mechanical action of the stomach. And there were the incomplete tables on digestibility of articles of food, both in the stomach and in vials. There was perhaps no border to this frontier.

{THIRTY-SIX}

ON THE MORNING OF THE 29TH OF SEPTEMBER, 1832, a coach rolled to a halt before the home of Samuel Beaumont in Plattsburgh, New York. The four horses at harness shook their heads and stomped their forelegs as the coachman gathered their reins and clucked his tongue to calm them. Behind him two penny travelers sat on the rooftop.

A young boy sprang up from his seat on an overturned bucket and ran forward to the coach. Before he could reach it, the door swung open so hard it slapped the coach side. The boy halted in midstep. The second door opened with slightly more care, and William Beaumont emerged, wincing momentarily from pain in his right knee. He smoothed his jacket front and took in the view of the house and its yard, cluttered with wheelbarrows, a wagon, several barrels and rakes of various dimensions. A chicken scurried around the house.

William Beaumont strode forward to the boy. His step was quick despite a limp. He was grinning.

"Here then, you're Young Willy?"

He placed a fond hand on the boy's tangled black hair.

The boy mumbled something like yes sir.

"I'm your uncle William, uncle of sorts. Your father and I are cousins. We've several trunks on top. Help the coachman with them. I'll tend to your aunt and cousins. Here you are, lad." He palmed the boy a coin.

He turned and swung down first his daughter Sarah, then Lucretia.

"Sarah, help your mother there with your brother."

Sarah reached into the coach and took the infant Israel into her arms. Lucretia was spinning around on the lawn so that the ribbons in her hair turned out as if on a May pole.

Beaumont took Deborah's hand and helped her from the coach.

"We're here."

She smiled.

"Yes we are."

The door to the house opened, and Samuel Beaumont stood at the worn threshold. In the fifteen years since their last reunion, he had lost considerably more hair. His pate was now bald and shiny. He'd also abandoned his business as a printer and become a physician.

THE ONLY MEN ENTITLED TO HAPPINESS

189

"Alice," Samuel called over his shoulder. "They're here."

Several children came racing out from behind him, and then came Alice. The yard was a crowd of children and adults, three excited dogs and a stack of trunks.

Samuel embraced his cousin. "You're two days early."

"We took a coach from Sackett's Harbor. The thing travels like lightning."

"Two more days then to enjoy your company. Have you eaten?"

They had not eaten since sunrise.

"Well, come in, come in. Let's gather your things and have some breakfast."

The children scrambled around the coach, laughing as they began to grab the trunks and bags, the little ones hefting them like sacks of flour while Alice attempted to direct them.

"You've a well-settled home here, Samuel," Beaumont said.

Samuel demurred.

"The place is in sorry shape."

"Has a man named Alexis St. Martin called? A French Canadian. Young fella. Have you heard any word?"

Samuel shook his head. "Called here?"

"Yes."

Samuel shook his head again.

Beaumont seemed to relax.

"Very well then, let's get Deborah and the children settled, and then I have to tell you about some business. Are you able to walk with me into town? Does a Jonathan Woodward still have his law offices and the American Fur Company an agent?"

Samuel was bemused.

"So quick to business, William. Yes, Jonathan thrives at his many ventures, and there is an agent at the dockyards. I have cases to call on, so we both have reason to venture to town."

WITHIN THE HOUR, the two Beaumont cousins were walking into the town of Plattsburgh.

Samuel, though younger by ten years, was shorter and stockier than his cousin and was soon breathing heavily as he kept up with William's long-legged stride. William was telling Samuel the story of Alexis St. Martin, his wound, the four experiments he'd published in the *Medical Recorder*, his return to Prairie du Chien and his successful negotiations with Dr. Lovell to secure a year's leave.

"I fully intend now to devote myself to the study of digestion and then to return to the army with Alexis as my particular charge."

"Here then? Deborah's last letter suggested that you all were moving here."

"We are. I'm sorry if it's all a bit confusing. The details only fell into place in the last few months. You can't imagine how difficult it's been to arrange for this leave, coordinate Alexis's arrival with my friends and contacts in the American Fur Company and arrange things for the coming year of study. I've waited seven years for this. Seven."

Beaumont stopped speaking and let out a small laugh.

"What is it, William?"

"I was counting the years. I'm mistaken. It has in fact been ten years since I met him when he was a lad. When I was stationed in Mackinac. Ten years almost to this month when I first realized that the wound was a unique opportunity. It seems so long ago. Like I was a different person."

"How long will this Alexis remain here?"

"What's that?"

"I was asking how long you shall be here, your plans of research."

"I trust only a few days. As soon as I have him here and some paperwork is done, we leave for Washington and then Paris."

"Paris? You can't be serious?"

"I am. It's the temple of medical research. There I shall make a study of him and exhibit him to the leading scientists. This will not only assure the research reflects the latest advances in physiology but also will open up the European market for the book. London is nearby. I shall likely take him there too. Moreover, the farther he is from his shrew of a wife, the better for my work. I learned many lessons all too well in my years in Prairie du Chien."

"Book?"

"Yes. I intend to publish the experiments in a book. *Experiments and Observations on the Gastric Juice and Digestion.* That's the working title, and it's outlined now to five sections: aliment, hunger, satiety and so on. The most important of which is digestion by the gastric juice. This shall be in every home in America. Everyone eats."

Samuel stopped walking. "Let's catch our breath."

The two men halted. Samuel took out his kerchief and wiped his brow and the smooth dome of his head. He looked at his cousin. "But what of Deborah and the children? You've just fathered your son Israel."

"I don't deny it's a sacrifice. But science demands this of me. The treasure that is that wound is deep and rich. And I could just as well be called off to war."

Samuel nodded to a passing laborer who greeted him as Dr. Beaumont. He looked at William. "Yes, of course. You could just as well be called to war."

"I shall need your help, Samuel. Your skills as a former printer. Can you help me locate a printer and see that the job is done right and at a fair price and that subscriptions are properly solicited? I've some money, but I'm not a rich man."

"I suppose I can, William, though I myself no longer am in the business, you know that. I still have the acquaintance of Francis Allen, the man I sold my business to. I can certainly introduce you to him and see that the negotiations are fair and proper."

Beaumont clasped his cousin's shoulders.

"That would be splendid, Sam, absolutely splendid. And see to it that he does not take this Connecticut farm boy for a fool and defraud me of my meager wealth? I've not a clue what this should cost. Only that I need to bang the drum loud for subscriptions."

"A clever Connecticut farm boy, I'd say. Your father always said you were the cleverest of the lot. Of course I shall help. There are several technical considerations, such as the paper and binding. Francis is reputable, but in the hands of a Boston or Philadelphia printer you might be out several hundred dollars before you have even your first copy in hand."

Beaumont embraced his cousin.

"Thank you. I can't tell you how much this means to me. The publication of this book shall be a triumph for American medicine. That's why I'm off to see Mr. Woodward. I must bind the ungrateful man to me, as a covenant servant of sorts. You see I've tried and failed to appeal to Alexis's duty, to his spirit of fairness, to industriousness. I've come to understand that his kind are not capable of such rational appeals. That was my folly. His are a more passionate, undemocratic kind who respond to pleasure and passion, and to power. Like an Indian. By God, it's been ten years, but on a clear day I can see hints of the shore."

"But are you sure it's China?"

"What?"

"China. When Italian and Spanish explorers came here they thought they were in China. That's what they desired. And look what they got."

JONATHAN WOODWARD's well-appointed office overlooked the town square and the Greek revival façade of the Clinton County courthouse. Woodward offered Beaumont a glass of sherry which Beaumont declined. They settled in chairs with the polished expanse of the split-top mahogany table between them. Benjamin Moores, Woodward's diminutive secretary, sat nearby with paper and pens.

They talked about the town, the sale of the Green family's United States Hotel and the auction of its contents.

"I've got one of their fish-eye mirrors here somewhere." Woodward glanced around the room. "Where is that? Had my eye on it since I first saw it. Oh yes, there." He pointed to the wall above a matching pair of side tables, their legs tapered and inlaid, their tops cluttered with decorative porcelains.

Beaumont recognized the piece. It was a gilded mirror with a fish-eye glass, on top of which was an eagle, its exaggerated talons clutching a bundle of arrows. It had once hung in the Greens' sitting room, where Beaumont called on Deborah to tell her the news of his posting as assistant surgeon at Mackinac Island. On that evening, they had been reading *Merchant of Venice.* An opportunity for both of us, he had told her. An opportunity to leave here and start again, together. As man and wife. It hasn't been easy for me.

Woodward was jovial, chatty and arrogant.

"I don't suppose you recognize the mirror, eh? The tales it might tell. I keep it there so I have an easy view of Benjamin at his desk."

The lawyer chuckled and twisted his gold signet ring. "Now then, Doctor, what business do you bring to me? Have you returned from the frontier with a fortune to invest? There are some splendid opportunities here now in Clinton County."

"Not exactly," Beaumont replied in an even tone. "I've need of an agreement to secure the cooperation of a man. The nature of the relationship and the work he is to perform, or rather permit me to perform, are unique. Let me explain from the beginning."

For the second time that day he told the story of Alexis St. Martin.

When he reached the end of the story, the squares of daylight cast through the western windows stretched long on the opposite wall. Woodward had stopped taking notes. His secretary Benjamin Moores was wide-eyed. The tall case clock seemed to resume its steady tick.

Woodward cleared his throat. "I thought perhaps you might come back with land or an interest in a mine, a share in the company."

Beaumont thought to tell him about his acres in Green Bay. They had increased in value some threefold. But he decided against it. It would only raise the lawyer's fee.

"You say an English doctor may take him? Caldwell?"

Beaumont nodded.

"English." Woodward pronounced the word slowly. "They nearly destroyed this town."

There was a kind of tension in the room. Exaggerated sounds came in from the square. Beaumont folded his elbows on the table top and leaned closer to the lawyer.

"You see, Jonathan, Alexis St. Martin is not like you and me. Despite *all* that I have done for him, at considerable personal expense and sacrifice, he remains ignorant of the many blessings and bounties I can bestow upon him as his benefactor. That is why I need an agreement that will clearly bind him to me for the purposes of science and scientific improvements. For the good that shall come of this for America and for him. I'd like to commission you to prepare that."

Woodward blinked several times and cleared his throat.

"You know, Doctor, agreements of indenture are now illegal in this state, but I could manage a kind of covenant that binds one man to another. Two free parties can make what is called a contract or covenant, much like a treaty between nations, between the Indian and the United States. It spells out the obligations of each to the other."

Beaumont nodded slowly and decisively. "That would be suitable," he said. "Quite suitable." He could scarce contain his pleasure.

Woodward blinked and then wiped his hand over his eyes and brow. "For how long?"

"One year. At least one year."

{THIRTY-SEVEN}

ON THE MORNING OF THE 19TH OF OCTOBER, William Beaumont met Alexis St. Martin in the dining room of the General Washington Tavern on the Plattsburgh Square. The two men dined quickly and silently. When they departed the inn, they crossed the square to Jonathan Woodward's office. There they met Woodward, Benjamin Moores and Paul Green, eldest son of Martha and George Green, apprentice to Benjamin and witness to this day's agreement. The five men gathered at the great table in Woodward's office. Woodward sat at the head. He adjusted his tiny spectacles, took up the pages and tapped them square.

"Gentlemen, let's begin."

Beaumont and Alexis made as if to stand.

Woodward looked up. "Please sit, gentlemen. There's no need to stand on ceremony."

Paul Green chuckled.

"Now then. If there are no questions as to the nature of the proceeding, I shall commence reading of the document. Mr. Green?"

Green folded his hands upon his lap and nodded. Woodward began reading.

"*Articles of agreement and Covenant, indented, made, concluded and agreed upon at Plattsburgh, in the County of Clinton and State of New York, the Nineteenth of October, in the year of our Lord one thousand eight hundred and thirty-two, between William Beaumont, Surgeon in the Army of the United States of America, of the one part, and Alexis St. Martin, Laborer, of Berthier, in the Province of Lower Canada, of the other part, to wit.*"

As Woodward pronounced each man's name, he gazed upon him and nodded, and each nodded in turn. Alexis removed his cap.

"*The said Alexis St. Martin, for the consideration herein mentioned, doth covenant, promise and agree to and with the said William Beaumont, his heirs, executors, administrators and assigns, by these presents in manner following—that is to say, that he, the said Alexis, shall and will for and during the full terms of one year, to begin and to be accounted from the date of these presents, serve, abide and continue with the said William Beaumont, wherever he shall go or travel, or reside in any part of the world, his covenant Servant, and diligently and faithfully, and according to the utmost of his power, skill and knowledge, exercise and employ him-*"

self in and do and perform such service and business matters and things whatsoever as the said William shall from time to time order, direct and appoint to and for the most profit and advantage of the said William, and likewise be just and true and faithful to the said William in all things and in all respects."

Woodward paused. He looked up over his glasses at Alexis. This section was his doing, based on his counsel that Alexis needed to be bound in a general manner, without condition to the task or purpose. "Think of it as an umbrella," he had explained to Beaumont. "It covers him entirely."

"Is that clear, Mr. St. Martin?"

"Yes sir," Alexis said quickly.

"There's more."

It was the section Beaumont had spent three days revising and rewriting in Woodward's office. "You'll have to help on this one, Doctor," Woodward had begged him. "It's out of my skill."

"And the said Alexis, for the consideration herein after mentioned, further specially covenants and agrees with said William that he, the said Alexis, will at times during said terms, when thereto directed or required by said William, submit to, assist and promote by all means in his power such Physiological or Medical experiments as the said William shall direct or cause to be made on or in the Stomach of him, the said Alexis, either through or by the means of the aperture or opening thereto in the side of him, that said Alexis, or otherwise, and will obey, suffer and comply with all reasonable and proper orders of experiments of the said William in relation thereto, and in relation to the exhibiting and showing of his said Stomach, and the powers and properties thereof, and of the appurtenances, and powers, properties, situation, and state of the contents thereof.

"It being intended and understood both by William and said Alexis that the facilities and means afforded by the wounds of the said Alexis in his side and stomach shall be reasonable and properly used and exhibited at all times upon the request or direction of said William for the purposes of science and scientific improvements, the furtherance of knowledge in regard to the power, properties and capacity of the human stomach . . ."

Now came the section the doctor and the lawyer had most struggled over. The doctor had insisted the terms precisely qualify the nature of the support Alexis would receive. "Only things necessary and in quantities that are reasonable and sufficient," he demanded. "I'm not some Indian agent handing out presents and treasury pap." He dismissed as naive the lawyer's plea that the requirement *to act to and for the most profit and advantage of the said William* was likely sufficient to limit the extent of Alexis's demands. "'For the most profit and *your* advantage, Doctor. You see then, he can't bankrupt you for a seven-course meal and a gold-fringed coat." But Beaumont was unmoved. "You don't know this Frenchman like I do," he insisted.

". . . And in consideration of the premises, and of the several matters and things

by the said Alexis to be performed, suffered and done as aforesaid, according to the true intent and meaning of the premises, and on condition that the said Alexis shall and does perform the same on his part, according to the true intent and meaning thereof, and not otherwise, the said William Beaumont doth for himself, his heirs, executors and administrators covenant, promise and agree to and with the said Alexis by these presents that the said William shall and will at all times during said term find and provide unto and for the said Alexis suitable, convenient rooms or house when with and in the service of said William, and also defray the necessary expenses and furnish the said Alexis good, suitable and sufficient subsistence, washing and lodging and wearing apparel when journeying with and at the request and direction of the said William. And also well and truly pay, or cause to be paid unto Alexis, his executors or administrators, the just and full sum of one hundred and fifty dollars . . ."

"One fifty," Alexis blurted out.

"Yes, one hundred and fifty American dollars total. Mr. Moores would you please show Mr. St. Martin the sum of his first installment?"

The secretary produced a leather wallet and opened its contents to display a packet of bills.

"And new boots?" Alexis gestured to his much-worn boots.

Everyone looked to Beaumont.

"If they are required, they shall be provided," he said simply.

"As I was reading, where was I?" Woodward scanned the page. "Here then." He resumed. *"The just and full sum of one hundred and fifty dollars lawful money of the United States of America in Manner following, to wit: the sum of forty dollars, parcel thereof, to be paid to said Alexis at or within one day after the execution of these presents, and the residue thereof, being one hundred and ten dollars, to be paid on personal application to said William, his executors or administrators at the expiration of the said term, which will be one year from the date hereof.*

"In witness whereof, as well the said Beaumont and the said Alexis St. Martin have hereunto set their respective hands and seals, the day and year first herein written, in the presence of each other and in the presence of Jonathan Douglas Woodward, Esquire, the subscribing notary public."

Woodward set the three pages down, one next to the other.

"So then, Doctor, Mr. St. Martin, unless there are questions, if each of you would make your mark we shall be done with this. Mr. Moores, would you be so kind?"

The secretary handed each man a pen.

Beaumont signed first, a quick decisive scratch of the pen, then slid the page over to Alexis.

Alexis held the pen awkwardly in his right hand. His grip resembled that of a child's when first learning to write.

"Right here, sir." Moores indicated Alexis's name on the document.

Between the words "Alexis" and "St. Martin" Alexis scratched a crooked, small letter "X."

"Is that your mark, sir?" Woodward asked.

Alexis nodded. He held the pen out for someone to take.

"Very well then. Mr. Moores, would you indicate that as such and then witness the document, followed by Mr. Green and then myself."

The three men made their signatures, and it was done.

Woodward rose from his chair and buttoned his coat over the great girth of his stomach.

"Well, gentlemen, I suppose I now pronounce you as Doctor and Covenant Servant. Good luck to you both with your work, such as it is. I shall be most interested to hear of its results."

Alexis spoke up. "Do I get my half?"

Moores stopped gathering the papers. Everyone looked at Alexis.

"Your half?" Woodward asked.

Beaumont spoke. His voice was oddly soft. "I think he means half of the agreement, to cut it in two pieces like an indenture. No, Alexis, there is not need to indenture this. It's an article of agreement and covenant that binds us together."

THE CLOCK IN THE PARLOR had struck two. Beaumont could tell by the measure of Deborah's breathing that she was awake beside him. He reached under the bed covers to embrace her and pulled himself close so that the arc of her back and soft rump fit snugly into the curve of his chest and waist. He stroked her thigh.

"I will miss you," he whispered.

They lay for some time listening to the steady cadence of the five children sleeping. Their daughters, Sarah and Lucretia, and Samuel's daughters, Emily and Constance, slept two girls to a bed. Israel was in his crib.

He embraced her tighter.

She crossed her arms over her chest. From the beginning, she had supported his preoccupations with Alexis, even after he was healed, even after he instigated a drunken scandal only to flee their home without thanks and then to come back to them with his angry wife in the muddy fever-infested swamps of Fort Crawford. And now he was going with the man for as long as a year, across an ocean to another world. Leaving her to raise their children in his cousin's crowded house.

"It's late," she whispered. "And you have to travel early."

"My dear," he murmured.

She lifted his arm and placed it on the mattress.

"I shall miss you too. Now sleep."

{THIRTY-EIGHT}

THREE DAYS AFTER THE MEETING in Joseph Woodward's office, before sunrise on a morning sufficiently cool that men's breath fogged and horses blew columns of steam like engines, a wagonette left the General Washington Inn carrying Alexis St. Martin, William Beaumont and their luggage to the Cumberland Bay dockyards, where they would board the steamboat *Phoenix*. By midmorning of the following day, they were on a flatboat on the Champlain Canal and by early evening, on a steamship from Albany traveling south on the Hudson River.

They arrived in the city of New York in the late afternoon and departed at dawn the following day from the Battery docks for New Jersey, then overland by coach to Baltimore. They stayed at inns, sharing rooms with other travelers, men with valises cut from carpet, lawyers on the circuit, traders and merchants. Men played cards and rolled die, drank and gossiped. In the mornings, they stood round the well in the tavern yard to shave and wash. For two days they shared coach with a garrulous man who called himself a journalist, spoke passable French and displayed an interest in Alexis until Beaumont requested he mind his business.

As they moved south, the accents of the people changed, grew longer, with words drawn out like chords on an old guitar. In Maryland they passed enormous farms, Georgian manor houses visible at the end of parallel lines of poplar trees, where gangs of Negroes mended fences and readied the brown fields for winter. These men looked up at them with expressions stolid and mute, then turned back to their monotonous labor under the gaze of the overseer with braided quirt and pistols. In Timonium, on the outskirts of Baltimore, they saw a slave auction presided over by an auctioneer who wore a blue silk top hat and sang out the virtues of his human wares. In Baltimore, they boarded the steamship *Meriwether Lewis*. On December 3, 1832, they docked at the Georgetown dockyards. William Beaumont and Alexis St. Martin had arrived in Washington City.

Alexis shivered against the chill of the wet wind as he stamped his feet, pulled his sleeves taut over his blue fingers and tucked his hands beneath his armpits. Beaumont commanded him to hurry along to the line of waiting carriages. The shift and flow of the crowds, the sight of men talking, arguing, making deals, all urged Beaumont to demand that the coachman

THE ONLY MEN ENTITLED TO HAPPINESS

199

hasten the journey to the Office of the Surgeon General of the United States.

THE TWO DOCTORS stood facing each other in the surgeon general's vast corner office, which was warm and dry, courtesy of a potbellied stove. The windows of the three-story hospital were visible across the clean-swept, white gravel courtyard.

"Dr. Lovell."

"Joseph. You must call me Joseph, William."

They shook hands, and then, in an instant, Lovell drew Beaumont closer, and they embraced.

Beaumont laughed. "All right then," he said over his mentor's shoulder. "Joseph."

Saying the name felt awkward, like calling his father Samuel.

"How long has it been?" Lovell asked. "I was thinking the other day of those many years since the war. Is it twenty? It is, isn't it?"

Beaumont knew the time to the month, as he had calculated it while reviewing his notebook during the journey. It had been nineteen years and eleven months since they had sat before the fire in the General Washington, near the Plattsburgh harbor, on a winter day so cold the teacups shattered if not properly warmed. Lovell had presented Beaumont with his worn copy of Antequil's *History*.

"Nearly twenty. We were at the camp in Plattsburgh."

"Along the Saranac River. I can see it all as if I just returned. And you were at the Battle of Plattsburgh, at Fort Moreau?"

Beaumont nodded.

Lovell sat and motioned for Beaumont to do the same. The lines of his long thin face had deepened into permanent creases, and the point of his chin seemed lengthened. His fine-curled hair had thinned and was graying at the temples; his thin lips were dry and near colorless.

"My years at a desk and the Washington summers have not been kind to my constitution. These last few months I've suffered from bilious colic. But I still have my wits." Lovell tapped his right temple. "I still meet veterans of that war. And look what's become of some of those men. General Scott. Colonel Taylor. And now you, Surgeon William Beaumont."

Beaumont smiled. "I'm just a humble surgeon."

Lovell chuckled.

"I always knew, William Beaumont, that you would make me proud. A man with your ambition and fortitude is destined to succeed in America. This country is designed for men such as you. I was just re-reviewing your quarterly reports from Prairie du Chien. It's splendid work you did on the frontier. You've no idea the motley quality of the reports I receive from the frontier. But it's Alexis who has my interest. Is he here?"

"Yes." Beaumont nodded to the door. "He's just outside. Shall I?"

"Not as yet, but I do very much want to see this gastric fistula. I trust you don't mind that I've made inquiries among friends and colleagues here and about. There's certain interest in the progress of your experiments. Some of the more learned congressmen are interested. Edward Everett of Massachusetts, have you heard of him? No? You shall, the man is a genius and a statesman. Brilliant orator. A future president, truly. I've known him since we were students at Harvard. He tutored me, or rather tried to tutor me, in Latin. But enough, I'm so pleased you're here. I have every expectation that your experiments will be of substantial value. I can hazard no better locale than here at the seat of our nation's power to unlock the secrets of the power of digestion."

Beaumont was grinning like a schoolboy.

"I expect I'll have a few weeks here before we depart for Paris. I've not inquired about our passage to France."

Lovell scanned his desktop as if searching for something. "Yes, that journey. Bear with me, but some things have happened since we last corresponded. I would have written you, but so much has been in flux, and I knew you were traveling here with all haste. It was not easy to secure your leave, as you know, given the continued hostilities along the frontier. Congress is not generous with funds. Your leave was reversed once, and on several occasions since then I have had to personally intervene to keep the special order granting it intact. The corps is spread thin."

Beaumont began to feel lightheaded. He remembered the younger and fitter Lovell, just two years after he'd graduated from Harvard's medical college, sitting at his desk at the hospital in Plattsburgh, patiently explaining to Beaumont that he had no doubts about Beaumont's skills as either a physician or a surgeon, but that to secure an appointment as a surgeon, the army required proof of training at a medical school.

Dr. Beaumont, Lovell had told him, I must counsel you to be patient. I see in you the flash of genius and the fire of ambition and a large natural talent. I can have you commissioned as a surgeon's mate, and in time, your promotion to surgeon will surely follow.

The Lovell who now sat before him reached for a paper. The long thin bones of his hands were visible under the thin skin.

"I think I have arranged for everything that you shall need to prosecute your experiments, housing and such and assure you there shall not be one iota of duty put upon you during this furlough. Mr. Pence, our librarian, is most eager to assist. He's a most capable man. If the ships were faster and the winter seas more temperate, I am sure you could make it to Paris, but I don't believe that six months will be sufficient time for you to journey to Paris and back."

"Six months?"

Lovell coughed as he set the paper down.

"I'm afraid that's all I've been able to secure for you. I can't manage one year. I'm sorry, William, I know this disappoints you, but this is the army. I assure you that you shall have all the resources you require here to guarantee the success of your work. If you'd like to remain in Washington, I've secured handsomely furnished quarters for you. Of course, I entirely understand if you wish to return to your family in Plattsburgh."

Without Lovell Beaumont knew he might be selling tonics from the back of a painted wagon. Without Lovell he might still be in Prairie du Chien, caught up in the ceaseless chaos of Indian wars.

"This is adequate, perhaps even more than adequate. Even during the journey south, I've managed substantial progress with my notes and reading. At Prairie du Chien, entire months passed without my having the time for experiments. The thought of having entire months, even just six, available for my experiments leaves me near giddy. I'm eager to begin work, and as soon as possible. Here in Washington."

Lovell smiled.

"Giddy perhaps, but I'm sure you'll remain standing. Excellent then. You have your rooms, the library is at your disposal, and I assure you your social calendar shall fast be crowded. You do have calling cards?"

"I do." Beaumont patted the pocket wherein he kept the wallet of newly printed cards.

"Excellent."

"I do have one request."

"Speak, please."

"As you know, I have sustained the care of Alexis at my own expense for several years now, since I first came to his aid really, in 1822 on Mackinac Island. After some months there, the leaders deemed him a common pauper and determined he was a drain upon their charity, limited as it was, and ordered him cast away in a bateau to fend for himself when the wound had not yet properly healed. I took the lad in to my home, and he was with us for some two years. In Prairie du Chien, I had charge not only of him but also of his wife and children. Food, clothing, bandages and now our travel here, his lodging and boarding. All these charges have come directly out of my own pocketbook. Several hundreds of dollars."

Beaumont paused and composed his request.

"It has occurred to me that were Alexis in the army, it would allow me to have him at the garrison here and elsewhere, secure some modest income for him over and above the generous income I provide him as part of our covenant, and cover his room and board."

"You wish Alexis to have a rank in the army?"

"Exactly. Perhaps in the commissary. Such light duties would make use of his skills as a common household servant."

Lovell regarded Beaumont. He drummed his fingers upon the desk. "Sergeant Alexis St. Martin. I might be capable of arranging that. How old is he?"

"Late twenties, I should think, more or less. Why do you ask?"

"In all this time, I've never known. Curious. Nonetheless, Lieutenant Cooper has charge of the commissary, and he's a decent fellow, though the lot he has charge of are an odd crew, veterans of the war some of them. I even recognize one from the hospital in Plattsburgh; fellow took a blow to the head that had him out for a day and a night. Left him a simpleton. Alexis must be as able-bodied as any of them. I think I can manage him a commission in the commissary."

"That would do just fine for Alexis. May I show you the wound now?"

"Yes, straightaway."

"He's not eaten since breakfast, so I'd expect that cavity empty. Hence I can demonstrate how I distill the gastric liquor with a simple gum elastic tube. Sometimes it flows quite freely, but not as well other times. I think not only appetite but also atmospheric conditions may influence the process."

THEIR QUARTERS WERE three rooms previously occupied by a recently deceased senior surgeon and his servant. Lovell's intervention had procured the space for Beaumont.

There was a sitting room with a mantled fireplace and space enough to accommodate a large table, bookshelves and several chairs. The view was the raked-gravel courtyard. The walls were decorated with two lithographs. *The Apotheosis of Liberty and Prosperity, 4 July 1814* showed allegorical figures of Liberty and Prosperity gazing down upon Colonel Scott and his staff in the aftermath of their victory against the British at Fort Erie. *American Vista* was a landscape. In the near distance stood a pair of Indians, each holding the bridle to his horse, as they gazed upon a herd of buffalo crossing the rolling plains below them. Attached to this sitting room were two bedrooms. The larger had a simple washbasin, dresser with mirror, wardrobe and a featherbed mattress on an iron frame. The other was narrow, with a sleeping pallet and washstand.

"These are adequate, more than adequate," Beaumont announced.

It was late in the afternoon when Beaumont and Alexis finished at Lovell's examination room. Beaumont and Lovell had passed two hours inspecting the wound, gathering gastric juice and sampling Alexis's meal of cold roast pork, bread and butter. Beaumont still carried in his vest pocket the warm vial of Alexis's gastric juice.

"Alexis, set my trunk of books there beside the shelf. I'll set up the sand bath and vials and other equipment here on the table which I'll also use for a desk. Let's move one of the chairs into your room so I can inspect the wound at bedside. I'll talk with Dr. Lovell about securing a small table for your meals and some kind of nightstand where I can keep equipment."

"*Ce que tu veux,*" Alexis muttered. "Why settle so much if we are only to travel again soon?"

"Alexis, please don't speak French."

"Paris?" he said dully. "*Ceci ce n'est pas Paris, non?*"

"There's been a change of plans. Unpack those books, and I'll explain. Just place them on the shelves, and I'll see to their order later. Mind their spines, some are delicate."

Alexis unbuckled the straps of the trunk and began to slowly unload its contents as Beaumont explained their new plans.

"But you said Paris?"

"Circumstances have changed. We must learn to live with them. I'd reckon this is a jot better than Prairie du Chien."

Alexis bent down to take up more books. Beaumont continued speaking.

"We're to stay here for several months. I'd expect until spring. In the meantime, I shall make inquiries about travel to Paris after the winter. I remain as anxious as you do to get there, but for now, we're here. It's a military matter that's out of our control. Besides, Alexis, I have some good news for you."

Alexis paused his labor and gazed expectantly at Beaumont.

"I've managed to secure you some additional income, over and above what you shall receive as part of our agreement. Twelve dollars a month salary and two dollars fifty for clothing and ten cents a day for subsistence. Do you like that?"

Alexis's fingers and lips were set in calculating motions.

"It's more than one hundred dollars a year, Alexis. One hundred forty-four, to be precise, not counting the food and clothing allowances. What say you?"

"When do I get it?"

"You'll have to talk with the paymaster in the commissary. Dr. Lovell thought it best you have the rank of a sergeant in the detachment of orderlies under Lieutenant Cooper. I agree with him. It's a sensible plan considering your status as a civilian among the military. The work is no more substantial than what you have done for me, as you shall be assigned as my orderly. When you finish with those books, you can unpack my clothes and settle yourself in your room. Then, you're to report to the commissary. It's just across the courtyard, the large brick building on the western side. The kitchens are there. I'm going to take care of some business, and tonight I shall dine with Dr. Lovell and his wife. Tomorrow, we start our work."

Beaumont inspected his watch, then he made to return it to the small pocket of his trousers, but then he stopped.

"One more thing, Alexis. Here."

He held out the watch on the palm of his hand.

"It's for you."

Alexis hefted it and slid it into the deep pocket of his trousers.

"Clip the chain to your belt loop. That way you won't lose it. Now that you have a timepiece, and I've another for myself, we won't have any troubles with missing observations. If you should retire before I return tonight, I'll see you first thing in the morning. Seven sharp. Don't forget, time is money."

{THIRTY-NINE}

NOW CAME DAYS OF EXPERIMENTS. Daily, before sunrise, Beaumont knocked on Alexis's door, leaned into the darkened room and announced "It's time." Then he stepped outdoors to record the temperature, the wind and precipitation. When he returned, Alexis lay waiting on his pallet, a small candle burning on the table, his chamber pot brimming, the tails of his shirt rolled up to expose the orifice. The croaking sound of hunger passed through the hole.

Beaumont set his lantern and supplies on the tabletop, sat on his stool and began the inspection of the gastric coats, both with and without his magnifying glass. Next, he measured the temperature in the cavity, removed the thermometer, wiped it clean with a soft flannel square expressly for this purpose and returned it to the felt-lined case. The he took up his gum elastic tube. Beaumont had only to hold out his hand and Alexis moved into position.

The tube inserted, he distilled the gastric juice, drop by clear drop, into a glass vial, each time Alexis complaining of the sinking feeling and darkening vision. This done, Alexis lay back as Beaumont corked the vial and stepped out to his worktable to set it beside others, some resting in one of his sand baths, the paper label of each vial bearing the number of its corresponding experiment. As Beaumont recorded his morning observations, Alexis washed, then dressed in his sergeant's uniform. Within an hour he returned with their breakfast and coal ration.

Hourly, Beaumont sampled and chronicled the contents and pace of digestion of every meal, sometimes on the quarter hour. Roast mutton, breast of mutton, bread, butter, potatoes, cold roast pork, beef boiled and broiled, raw radishes, boiled chicken, wheat bread, hard-boiled eggs, pints of coffee. Some meals he simply let Alexis eat, while others he took samples, weighing out two to four drachms of a portion of that day's meal and wrapping it in a muslin bag suspended into the hole. Still other samples he placed into the vials in the sand bath.

Within a week, it was evident Alexis was drinking, some nights into a shuffle-footed, wall-scraping intoxication. Beaumont neither said a word nor acted to intervene. Every morning and at all hours until after dinner, the man submitted to examinations and observations without protest, and the effect of ardent spirits on the cavity and the process of digestion yielded excellent results. It was the kind of data Beaumont needed to educate the public on the hazards of spirituous liquors, the necessity of Temperance.

Between observations, he worked at his desk like an explorer deep in a valley described by mountains of books he gathered from Mr. Pence's library. He read Magendie and Abernathy. Philip's treatise on indigestion. The chapters on digestion in Dunglison's textbook. He copied out passages and made a table whose columns and rows fast multiplied with theories, and with this table he could reckon how some theories converged but then others diverged.

His synoptic table showed these scientists to be like the fanatical preachers of New York State, splintering each other's dogma with the ax of a new theory, then gathering and chopping the facts to fit a new theory. Each seemed equally correct, and each seemed equally deficient. Reaumur retrieved his gastric juice from sponges he forced buzzards to swallow. Young studied frogs and his own vomit. Spencer used dogs. What none of them possessed was the plain and unvarnished truth, unfettered by the heirlooms of theory and the crude observation of lesser animals. None of them had Alexis and his endless supply of gastric liquor.

In time, their rooms became a factory of discovery, and Alexis was fully transformed. Beaumont came to see only the experiments at hand. Alexis's thin body became like a patent machine centered at the puckered hole. The variations in experiments were as numerous as every act, every motion, every mood and meal his Frenchman experienced. He placed masticated portions of food into a vial of gastric juice and into another of pure water and still a third vial with unmasticated food into saliva he ordered Alexis to spit up. Then he ordered Alexis to cradle these vials in his armpits as he performed his chores or took his customary walk from their barrack to the dockyard and back. Beaumont allayed Alexis's sense of hunger and stopped the croaking noises caused by the motion of air in the stomach and intestines by putting directly through the aperture three and a half drachms of lean boiled beef. The next day he introduced eight ounces of lukewarm beef and barley soup through a tube, with a syringe.

Scientific efficiency governed their every action. Some days, they exchanged only a few words. Nothing was wasted. All was recorded. Days of Alexis's sullen laziness afforded observations of the effects of total lassitude upon the pace of digestion, while his anxious restlessness demonstrated the effects of vigorous exercise and appetite. Beaumont charted the course of moods: anger over a delayed meal, anger over the insertion of the muslin bag through the tender margin of the hole and into the cavity. Costiveness slowed the pace of digestion and was relieved by calomel applied directly into the aperture. He recorded days when Alexis's tongue was dry and furred with a thin, yellowish coat, his dark eyes heavy and countenance sallow. The membrane of the protruded portions of the stomach was a mirror image of the tongue.

Callers came to see the man with the hole in his side: several physicians in the surgeon general corps; Dr. Henry Hunt, President Jackson's physician; three professors from Columbia Medical College; a Very Right Reverend of the Episcopal Church and close friend of Lovell's; a reporter from the *National Intelligencer.*

By the end of the third week, Beaumont had recorded thirty experiments in his notebook and had set upon the mantelpiece a tidy stack of two dozen calling cards, along with an invitation to a reception for a recently appointed undersecretary of the navy, another for a tea hosted by the wife of General Scott, and the most cherished—President Andrew Jackson's Christmas Ball.

THE JAM OF CARRIAGES AND GIGS lined Pennsylvania Avenue a mile from the White House. Many guests decided to simply leave their vehicles and walk the distance, passing a detachment of marines with bayonets fixed. They'd been called out to maintain order among the rowdy crowds of laborers and hangers-on who had come up from the Georgetown docklands and swirled like a horde of insects in the feeble yellow glow of the oil lamps lining the fog-blanketed length of Pennsylvania Avenue. A fight nearly broke out between a group of laborers and another of free Negroes. The air smelled of the grease of cooking fires. An elderly man paused to wipe the mist from his spectacles. Crowds gathered on the White House lawn, passing bottles, singing Irish carols and demanding, and in due course receiving, their fair share of the party. This was not simply a Christmas celebration but also a celebration of the reelection of President Andrew Jackson and his new vice president, Martin Van Buren.

Inside the ballroom, the string and brass band created a general din that amplified the noise of the crowd so that many had to shout to be heard. The heat grew oppressive; red-faced men unloosened their cravats and flapped their jackets like great flightless birds; the ladies smartly fanned themselves and dabbed their powdered brows. The servants threw open the doors and windows.

The ostentatiously victorious Southern Democrats slapped each other's backs, journalists and judges wandered everywhere, and a few dour Northern Whigs sullenly sipped punch. News and gossip were heard everywhere.

"Will the Negro rise up?"

"Wasn't the Thorntons' ball grand?"

"Calhoun is finished."

"They no longer serve the best turtle soup at the Epicurean Eating House."

"Look at the poonts on that girl."

There were diplomats in formal dress with the emblems of their nation's high honors and ceremonial swords with gold-braided hilts and silver scabbards, officers with chests thick with colored medals and crossed by crimson sashes. Children ran about with candy sticks and small white frosted cakes topped with yellow raisins. Some discovered that in stocking feet they could slide along the dance floor as if it were a winter pond. The servants carried in buckets to replenish the punch bowls, set silver platters piled with cakes and sandwiches on a table as long as a carriage. Young men lurked near the mistletoe.

Despite this activity there was a distinct sense of power in the room, centered on President and General Andrew Jackson. Jackson was dressed in black and buttoned high to the Adam's apple, like a parody of a severe Northern Whig or Unitarian minister, his golden hair swept back, pomaded and combed smooth, as if burnished by the glow of his victory. He stood beside a conifer twice his height which was decorated by tiny white candles and red ribbons. The pace of the receiving line to greet the president was so slow that people cut in and out of the line. After one hour of gradually advancing, Dr. William Beaumont stepped forward to shake the hand not of the Hero of New Orleans but of his vice president, the Little Magician, Martin Van Buren. The man was stiff and short as a stump.

"Merry Christmas, Mr. Vice President."

"Merry Christmas to you too, sir."

The vice president scanned the symbols of Beaumont's dress uniform, nodded at the caduceus and praised him for his service to the surgeons corps.

"Surgeon General Lovell is a most able officer," he declared.

"Yes indeed he is, Mr. Vice President, and a great friend and colleague as well. We've known each other since the War of 1812. I expect he is somewhere among this gathering. You know, Mr. Vice President, you and I share a bond as fellow New Yorkers. You from Kinderhook and I from Plattsburgh. I'm William Beaumont, surgeon in the corps."

"A fine city in a great state. Do you know my good friend Francis Woodward?"

Beaumont nodded vigorously. "A good man."

"Such a pleasure, Doctor. Do let my secretary know if there is anything I can do to assure the success and comfort of your stay in our capital. I take special care of my fellow New Yorkers. Governor Throop, himself, he is somewhere among us."

Beaumont produced one of his newly printed calling cards.

"I have the honor to be stationed at the Naval Yard under Surgeon General Lovell's command to complete a study of digestion upon a patient I've cared for, for some ten years now. Dr. Lovell and I anticipate that the results shall be most informative for the health of all Americans. Dietetics is essential to a robust constitution."

Van Buren nodded solemnly as he pocketed the card and offered Beaumont one of his own.

"Most interesting. Progress in science is, as in commerce, essential to the success of our great American experiment."

Beaumont let the flow of the receiving line carry him away from the vice president. He could scarcely contain his thrill. He downed a cup of sweet punch in one gulp, stepped into the chill of the evening and loosened his collar as he gazed at Van Buren's calling card. The card of the vice president of the United States of America was his. Men such as this could see in this son of a failed Yankee farmer the promise of America's progress along a new frontier.

Several guests mistook Beaumont in his dress uniform for an army officer and asked him about the great chief Blackhawk and the war that bore his name. When they discovered that he was a medical officer, some retreated to refill their punch glasses, others told tales of their fevers, aches, and pains. A few asked about the purpose of his stay in Washington. In time, he fell into lecturing to a group of seven guests.

"Spices, alcohol, none of these things are digested and thus possess no nutritive properties. They simply pass out of the stomach and into the circulatory system, surely to do harm elsewhere. You see, they don't coagulate, so there is no way that the gastric juice can act upon them. But milk. Milk is, I tell you, the ideal substance for digestion; it readily coagulates upon mixing with the gastric juice. There should be sufficient cows in every fort and garrison."

Several of the company gathered before him gazed at their punch glasses. Two men, dressed in the high style with striped trousers buttoned high to the waist and colorful frock coats, clinked their cups and drained them.

The young man in a salad green jacket leaned forward. "And what of cheese?"

Beaumont shook his head.

"One might think so, sir, but consider its closeness of texture and its large portion of fat. Both are not readily amenable to easy action of the gastric juice. Thorough mastication is essential. Absolutely essential."

"Mastication," the young man repeated.

An elderly man with a puckered face turned en bloc to a frail woman who stood beside him.

"Did you hear that, Emily? Cheese is not proper for the diet. Perhaps we should talk with Bessie? She's our cook," he said to Beaumont. "A very capable Negress. Cheese is often served at our table."

Two ample-bosomed ladies who stood in the periphery blushed and hid their smiles behind the needlepoint-ornamented crests of their silken fans.

❦{FORTY}❧

AFTER THIRTY-EIGHT DAYS OF CONTINUOUS EXPERIMENTS and observations upon Alexis, as Beaumont was recording experiment number fifty-seven, Dr. Lovell called with a visitor, a slender man whose curly red hair was cut close like that of a Roman senator, his cheeks flush from the cold. His frock coat was the customary gentlemen's black, but its details displayed signs of wealth. Gold buttons, a silk lining. Lovell introduced the man.

"This is a surprise, I know, William. But I have the honor of introducing Dr. and Professor Robley Dunglison from the University of Virginia. Gentlemen."

Robley Dunglison was personal physician to Thomas Jefferson, a physiologist and author of *Human Physiology.*

"Dr. William Beaumont," he said as he extended his hand. He was an Englishman. "Joseph wrote to me some months back that you were to be in Washington City. It is an honor now to stand here in your laboratory."

Beaumont stammered.

"The honor, the honor is, sir, rather mine."

"It's mutual, then. You must pardon my calling without proper invitation, but I had reason to be in the city, and until the frosty weather of the last week, the muddy roads from Charlottesville gave little hope for swift passage until spring. When they froze, I simply decided to travel with all haste to Washington."

Dunglison surveyed the cluttered room.

"You've assembled a most handsome laboratory here. Truly."

Lovell spoke up. "William, as you know, Dr. Dunglison is one of the principal proponents of the theory of digestion as a chemical process. His work in this area is most thoughtful."

"Here, here," Beaumont interjected.

"Robley, I should note that it was an error by the editor of the *Medical Recorder* that my name is ascribed to those four experiments. The credit is entirely William's."

"Of course," Dunglison said. "I had every intent to reference the work in the first edition of *Human Physiology,* but the journal was mislaid and I could not refer to it in time. A deadline loomed. Publishers are like wives when their minds are made up."

The three men chuckled.

"But I vividly recollect the results. They confirmed the experiments Spallanzani made at *l'hôpital de la charité* on a female with a fistulous opening into the stomach."

He gazed over to the worktable with its ordered arrangement of vials of gastric juice, the sand baths and notebooks.

"I see that since your first experiment you have doubtless instituted others."

Beaumont stepped over to the table and took up one of the vials containing clear juice. He held it up before them like some jewel and turned it so it refracted the light of a sunbeam.

"Herein, Doctor, is the gastric liquor. I distilled this some two weeks ago. It is as it was when it first flowed from the cavity. Observe."

He removed the cork and passed the vial before his nose, agitated it a bit and waved the flat of his free hand to encourage the odor to his nose, then touched the tip of his pinky into the fluid and onto his tongue. He handed the vial to Dunglison, who repeated these same maneuvers, then to Lovell. The three men were like dedicated oenophiles sampling a new vintage. When Dunglison tasted the liquid, he winced.

"It is most certainly acidic."

"And entirely free of putrefaction," Beaumont insisted. "I've a vial I've kept since my first experiments in Mackinac, and it remains as this one. Clear, free of putrefaction and acidulous in taste. And look here."

He took up another vial. It had a nut brown sediment at its bottom.

"You see here. Three ounces of broiled breast of mutton, four ounces of wheat and corn bread. It has been in here since the 26th of December."

He looked closer at the label. "No, forgive me. Experiment number 28. Just one moment."

He set the vial down, put on his spectacles and consulted his notebook.

"Number 28! Experiment number 28. That's December the 27th. Not the 26th. You'll see, as in all others the sediment that remains is entirely without evidence of putrefaction. Please."

Beaumont passed the vial to Dunglison, who uncorked it and performed the same maneuvers as he had with the first.

"Perhaps less acidulous."

"Precisely. The chemical nature exhausts itself, but the addition of more fresh liquor readily recommences digestion. There clearly is a proper ratio of aliment to gastric liquor. You see the origins of indigestion when too much aliment, especially aliment that is not properly masticated, passes too quickly into the cavity."

Lovell nodded. Dunglison simply gazed at the vial.

"So have you proven that saliva is not the sole agent in digestion as Montegre supposes but merely an adjuvant?"

"Montegre is plainly mistaken," Beaumont insisted.

"He is," said Dunglison. "Might I see this French boy of yours?"

"Of course." Beaumont stepped over to the door to Alexis's bedchamber. "Alexis," he called.

"Is he here?" Lovell asked.

"He's here. He naps frequently. But now he's due for an inspection of the cavity. This morning he dined on fatty pork and bread, though I should expect by now the cavity is entirely empty."

Beaumont rapped a knuckle on the door.

"Alexis, we have a visitor." He swung open the door. "Alexis, a doctor from Virginia is here. Dr. Robley Dunglison."

"*Une moment.*" There was the sound of a bedframe creaking.

"English, Alexis," Beaumont muttered as he turned from the door. "Grant him a minute to awaken."

WITHIN AN HOUR, Alexis lay shirtless on a table. They had moved his pallet out into the sitting room that doubled for Beaumont's laboratory as there was not sufficient room for all four men in Alexis's narrow bedchamber. The coal fire was low but the room still dry and warm, and the three doctors had their shirtsleeves rolled up above their elbows. Dunglison's spectacles had slipped to the tip of his thin nose. The pleasantries and courtesies of the morning had long vanished. The issue was the influence of the muslin bag on the course of digestion.

"Yes, yes, yes," Dunglison repeated. "I take your point, Dr. Beaumont. I do. I do. But enough about the muslin bag."

Dunglison had a manner of noting a point by gesturing with his left pinky like some miniature wand, touching it to his chin, pointing, and that skinny digit was decorated with a thin ring of gold that held the Dunglison family crest. His accent had become sharper. He leaned over and took up the notebook, turning the pages as he spoke.

"What *precisely* is your hypothesis?"

"My hypothesis?"

"Yes, hypothesis. What you set out to prove."

Beaumont stiffened.

"That digestion is a chemical process. That it is not accomplished by putrefaction and grinding but a chemical process. That is my hypothesis."

Dunglison turned several pages of the notes. He looked at Beaumont over the rims of his spectacles. "You have proven it. You proved it even with your few experiments in Mackinac many years ago. That, sir, is brilliant. *Brilliant.*"

"Thank you, Doctor." Beaumont's voice was hardened.

"My appeal to you is that you pursue observations by means of rigorous hypothesis testing, and, I might also add, it would be of value to standardize your methods as much as possible. It is all very well to say that digestion is a chemical process, but even better to say what that chemical is. I take it you're new to science, in particular to chemistry. Most days, if not all, you have the coffee measured out—a pint, I see—I assume he took it without any milk or sugar? And yet the bread, the toast, the butter, the sausages, none of them are measured or weighed. Hence your observations of the ratio of aliment to gastric liquor are not as sound as they might be. As a kind of diary of digestion this is most useful—I had a great-aunt in Sussex who kept such a thing, hers was of course cruder in its way—and yet I think that if you're to subject a man to daily inspections, multiple times in a day, you ought at least to have clear standards in your methods."

Dunglison exhaled heavily. He looked over at Alexis and then leaned in closer to Beaumont. He lowered his voice. "With all due respect, Doctor, it would balance the sacrifice you've subjected your lad to, I should think. There's just so much you can expect the man to take. There has to be some rational end to this work. I'm most willing to offer you some guidance in these matters."

Beaumont swallowed hard.

"I do most value your suggestions. I'm just a humble inquirer after the truth, of course, with neither the training nor position of a scientist such as yourself. Much like any explorer in a new land, I trust in my own eyes and ears and taste. To speak plainly, sir, and with all respect due to a man of your scientific stature and education, I think that the shackles of theory have been just that upon the field of physiology."

Dunglison set down the notebook.

"Dr. Beaumont, please take no offense at these remarks."

"None taken."

"And none intended. I only wish to see this most excellent work have the fullest impact upon the field. To finally establish that digestion is a chemical process, not fermentation or grinding. To settle the role of saliva as well. Your observations of the motions of the coats in the pyloric region are astounding, akin to the thrill Vespucci must have experienced when first gazing upon the coast of the New World. But what you need to learn is chemistry so that you might discover what this chemical is that makes the process possible.

"If you publish only what you have here, I do fear that the essential message shall be lost." Dunglison held the thumb and forefinger of his right hand before his face as if to secure some tiny and precious thing. "Focus, focus, focus, Dr. Beaumont," he pronounced. "Lead them to the light of the truth. That, sir, that, will assure you your place in the scientific pantheon."

"Here, here."

It was Lovell.

Dunglison faced Beaumont.

"And do consider organizing your results by theory and method. In your book, I should think that would be most useful."

IT WAS EARLY EVENING when Beaumont escorted Dunglison and Lovell to a carriage in the swept gravel courtyard. The image of the carriage, then its creak and rattle along the drive and finally the glow of its running lanterns vanished entirely into the gloom. The temperature had plummeted and a damp and cold wind blown in from the north. Men crossed the yard with a kind of odd swing to their torsos as they kept their bare hands tucked under their arms or stuffed deep into the pockets of their trousers. Beaumont shivered.

In these last few weeks he had seen the contours of his fame more clearly than ever, imagined that this hospital's entrance might one day bear his name etched upon its frieze. But Dunglison's words cast him into anger and despair. He had overheard the Englishman whisper to Dr. Lovell as the men settled into the carriage, "A raw talent, to be sure, but it was your Mr. Franklin who said that he who teaches himself has a fool for a master, or some such truism. I really do wish you'd summoned me sooner. Truly."

The bitter memories of his years at war returned. Memories of himself, the apprentice-trained surgeon's mate, speaking up at conferences and the university-trained surgeons ignoring him, mocking him.

He began walking across the courtyard. He missed Debbie, Sarah, Lucretia. Israel. His son. His only son. Debbie had written of the boy's temper, of how she wished her husband would be done soon with the book and return to them. He spat.

"To come this far, so near the summit of my ambition, only to turn back, to surrender the glory, because some arrogant, some jealous, some *English physiologist* pretends he can intimidate me into sharing the credit. Diary of digestion! Bah! Alexis is mine. His wound is *mine*. Every ounce of his gastric liquor is mine. *Mine!* To hell with the Englishman," he said loudly enough that a passing soldier turned and begged Beaumont's pardon.

When Beaumont returned to the cold gray room, Alexis lay as the doctors had left him, flat out upon his cot, his skinny arms folded over his chest. Beaumont stood for a moment and regarded the slow rise and fall of his arms, then shook his head and sat at his worktable.

"You should have hit him," Alexis said.

Beaumont looked up from his notebook. His reflection in the darkened window gazed back at him.

"What?"

"Hit him. For insulting you."

"You don't know what you're talking about."

Alexis snorted.

"It was a scientific discussion. I wouldn't expect you to understand such things," Beaumont said curtly.

"I don't. But I'm not stupid. He made a fool of you."

Beaumont turned to face Alexis. The Frenchman had not changed his position.

"Why don't you get up and carry your pallet back to your room?"

"That Englishman was rude. They always are. In Canada, they treat us French like shit."

Beaumont turned a page of his notebook.

"Your pallet, Alexis, return it to your room, and then set the chairs in proper order. I'd like you here at seven before you eat. That will be all."

Alexis slowly swung his legs over the edge of the pallet and sat up. As he did so gas emitted from his fistula with the long, drawn-out, wet sound of flatus. He grunted with disgust.

"*Merde,*" he muttered. He rose and rearranged his blouse, sniffing its armpits.

"You and me, *Docteur,* we are of a lot who is alike. Two farmer's boys trying to make it in the big and the bad world. I'm running out of money, by the way. Two dollars, please."

"At the pace you spend, Alexis, you shall be through your allowance well before your next payment is due."

"And you will then have me to starve, sir?" Alexis gestured with his pinky in a perfect mockery of the English physician.

Beaumont did not see this gesture. He remained hunched over his notebook, the words now swimming before his eyes.

"That's enough, Sergeant," he barked. "You have your orders."

❧{FORTY-ONE}❧

BY FEBRUARY, BEAUMONT HAD PENULTIMATE DRAFTS of the chapters on aliment, hunger and thirst, satisfaction and satiety, mastication and the appearance of the villous coat. The concluding chapter's list of inferences numbered thirty-five. What remained was the chapter he judged the most important: on digestion by the gastric fluid. The meeting with Dunglison had convinced him he needed a chemist to help him identify the chemicals in the gastric liquor. And he believed he had found that man.

He had met the Swedish ambassador at Congressman Edward Everett's dinner party two weeks before. In addition to the ambassador, the guests included the district attorney of Washington, Francis Scott Key; Senator Henry Clay; two Prussian brothers who ran a bank; a scholar of philology; an ancient Congregationalist minister; and Surgeon General Lovell.

Everett, a classmate of Lovell's from Harvard, led the conversation from the head of his sumptuously laid table, presiding like a tutor; he directed the conversation from Goethe's essays on optics, to a mediocre performance of Mozart's piano sonatas by the touring French pianist Monsieur Delmar, to President Jackson's obduracy over the national bank and the ascendancy of Jackson's brain, the Little Magician Martin Van Buren. As at all gatherings of Washington's wise and connected, Democrat and Whig, the remarks—both high and low—made reference to the problem of the Negro, both free and enslaved, and the amalgamation of the races. Everett and Key were among the leaders of the American Colonization Society, newly revived by the slave rebel Nat Turner's uprising in Southampton County, Virginia. The society's mission was to relocate all Negroes back to their native Africa.

It was not until dessert that the congressman asked Beaumont about the experiments he was performing. Beaumont flushed till his ears were warm and his armpits damp. He had hardly spoken all evening. He began the story of the man with the hole in his side. Several guests set down their silver spoons. The philologist began rubbing his abdomen. Senator Clay was wide-eyed. The minister roused from his slumber. They all wanted to know how Alexis came to acquire his wound and the manner of his miraculous recovery. Among all the guests, the ambassador showed the most interest. He was especially curious about the chemical properties of the gastric juice.

The ambassador was a tall and broad-shouldered man with a low and commanding voice. "In Stockholm," he explained, "we have the Royal Caroline Institute where the chemist Jons Jakob Berzelius presides. I have every expectation that Professor Berzelius would be most appreciative of the opportunity to apply his talents to ascertain the chemical components of the mysterious juice. Could you get me a specimen?"

At the close of Everett's dinner, the congressman quoted Francis Bacon's belief that knowledge is power and proclaimed Alexis St. Martin an American Experiment. "A book on dietetics comes at a most propitious time," he said, "what with Dr. Sylvester Graeme and his healthful cracker and the spread of the temperance and vegetarian movements among even the lesser classes. You, sir," Everett summarized, "have gathered great riches from the wilds of America, and we must keep these riches in America."

NOW THE TWO MEN sat in the ambassador's study. The inlaid card table between them was set out with a full tea service. The china displayed the royal crest of Sweden; the spoons were made of gold.

"Would you consider bringing your Frenchman to Sweden?" the ambassador asked.

"Most certainly yes. I had intended to travel to Paris, but my furlough of study was truncated such that I was forced to remain here, in Washington City. But I remain committed to bringing this great knowledge to Europe."

The ambassador nodded as he chewed a piece of cake. "A voyage made in the spring would have you in Stockholm around the time of the summer solstice. There are days when the sun never sets."

Beaumont visited with the ambassador for another hour. The man was eager to hear stories of the American West. He had once met Captain Hitchcock while visiting Clamorgan's Italian Baths in St. Louis. Hitchcock and he shared a fascination with Dante's *Divine Comedy*. As Beaumont returned to the Naval Hospital in the evening, his mind was all afire. The damp streets reflected the glow of the gas lamps like scarcely visible suns through the smoke and clouds at Prairie du Chien. People walked hunched up in miserable resignation to the penetrating wet cold, but Beaumont needed to throw off his blanket and cracked open the window of his carriage to allow the night air to cool him.

He had devoted two weeks to collecting the gastric fluid he gave the ambassador. Within the fortnight, a ship would leave with the container in a diplomatic pouch. By summer, he would have the results of Berzelius's analyses. With the mysterious substance in the gastric juice identified, that most important section of the book could be done, and by winter the book published.

He would put copies into the hands of the leaders of Washington—Joseph Lovell, Vice President Van Buren, Senator Clay, Francis Scott Key,

Congressman Everett, and Secretary Cass—and these men would, in turn, use their influence to see to it that Congress voted him compensation for his expenses and a stipend to continue his research. They all knew each other, and now they knew William Beaumont. Within a year, he would travel with Alexis to Paris, then to Stockholm and the court of King Karl Johan. Perhaps these countries would also see the value of supporting studies on the man with the hole in his side.

BEAUMONT WORKED DAILY, often past midnight, pausing for a quick meal, sometimes nodding off at his desk until Alexis awakened him, stumbling drunk and whistling into his room.

At the end of March Beaumont and Alexis prepared to depart Washington. The necessary papers were secured for their travel to Plattsburgh and to drop Sergeant Alexis St. Martin from the rolls of Lieutenant Cooper's detachment of orderlies. His orders now were to be subject to Surgeon William Beaumont's orders. The idleness that attended a move, when all possessions are packed, annoyed Beaumont. He simply could not stop working. There was so much still to do.

Alexis was slouched in an armchair with his boots propped up on the edge of the windowsill and his arms folded behind his head. He was gazing out at the detachment of orderlies idly raking the gravel square. Beaumont had been telling him about their travels for the coming weeks: New York, New Haven to visit with Dr. Silliman, then Boston and the doctors at Harvard College, and by June, July at the latest, Plattsburgh, where Alexis would stay at Samuel Beaumont's along with William and his family. Deborah had consented. Alexis listened with neither remark nor question.

"One year from now, Alexis, we shall set sail for Paris."

Alexis looked up at Beaumont. "You said that last year."

"Is that the way you talk with Lieutenant Cooper? I'm telling you now, things have changed. Important people have finally taken notice. Dr. Silliman is one of the nation's leading chemists. We're going to be famous."

"And?"

"Don't be difficult. Show some gratitude, perhaps? They see the value in my experiments. Your wound has paid you well and will continue to do so. That is my covenant to you."

Alexis leered. His lips moved, but no words came. He swung his legs down from the sill and rocked onto his feet. He gazed at the print of Colonel Scott victorious at Fort Erie.

Beaumont followed Alexis's gaze. "What is it?" he asked.

"What?"

"I said, what is it? What's wrong?"

Alexis shrugged. "Nothing is wrong. We're packed and ready to go. Just as you ordered."

Alexis was now gazing upon Beaumont's worktable.

"Why are you so sullen?" Beaumont insisted. "What are you doing? Put that down, Sergeant. That's an order."

Alexis was holding one of the vials of Beaumont's latest experiments on artificial digestion. The liquid within was the color of strong tea and the layer of sediment as dark as molasses. Alexis turned the vial slowly to and fro.

"This is not quite what I expected. I thought it would be clearer now."

Beaumont sighed. He reached out and set his right hand square upon Alexis's shoulder, but Alexis shifted. The hand dropped.

"How did you—when did you—when did you know that this would be like this?"

"What are you trying to say?" Beaumont snapped.

"When did you know that I had this, this gift?"

Beaumont's eyes narrowed. "What's your question?"

"Is that why you came back to rescue me from the shop?"

"That is a silly question, an insult as well. I tried by all means to heal that closed, all means, offered even to sew it closed, but you refused." Beaumont directed his index finger to within inches of Alexis's face. The man did not flinch. "It's obvious of course, now and in light of the knowledge I have subsequently discovered, that the wound would never close. That it will never close. The action of the gastric juice upon the wound is both what saved you and also what keeps the wound open. The juice worked like muriatic acid to cleanse the wound, but also it kept the vital tissues from growing and in time scarred them into place. The sutures of surgery would have been eaten away, the hole become even bigger. You just have to accept the way you are. Your curse and your blessing. You shall have that hole for the rest of your life. Make the best of it. That's what I've been trying to do all these years."

Alexis nodded. "Once upon a time, I thought these things were all planned, by God. I thought you were all that I needed. Sometimes now I wish you'd let me die."

Beaumont was indignant. "Don't talk such nonsense. It was an accident. An act of God. Such things happen in life, you know that." He paused and reached his right hand out again, this time with tenderness.

"Alexis, you have so much to live for," he said. "You just have to make the best of things. Think of your family."

"I was just an *enfant* then. Mine was a simple prayer to live, and now see what has become of me."

"Alexis, congressmen, senators, the vice president of the United

States—Old Kinderhook himself—leading chemists, physicians, great men, men who one, two, even three centuries from now will occupy the pantheon of American history, they all know about you. You. They all await this book with *eager* anticipation. You and I, we're bound together to make this world a better place. I accept that responsibility and have made it worth your while."

Alexis simply stared out the window. "My father was a drunkard who cast me from his house."

Beaumont looked back at the progress of the orderlies with their rakes on the gravel. They had now stopped their work and were leaning on their rakes, talking and jesting.

"And mine, Alexis, was a stubborn Yankee farmer with a wooden plow who couldn't see the right side of a profitable bargain even if it smacked him on the side of his proud face. Remember, Alexis, I know what it's like to be hungry. We two farmer's boys share something in common."

The two men gazed out the window. Alexis began to chuckle. Two of the orderlies were now winging handfuls of gravel at the third, who gestured obscenely with the handle of his rake and danced a kind of jig.

"I remember that first day, when I awoke. I was alone and it was dark, and I thought I had died and that perhaps I was in Heaven. Then I felt the pain, and I knew I must still be alive. What became of the old man who told the funny stories? Elijah?"

"Elias. Elias Farnham. He was still there when we departed Mackinac."

"And the ladies with their books. Madame Sally. I still think about her and her red-covered book."

Beaumont regarded Alexis. "Why, why did you flee me in Mackinac?"

Alexis shrugged. "To be free, I suppose."

Beaumont exhaled slowly through his nose. "That's absurd. I freed you of your indenture. We struck a deal in my office at the hospital. You do realize that if we had continued that work then in Mackinac, you and I now could have long returned from Paris, and be well settled now at one of the universities, and you with a good wage? We'd never have suffered the likes of Prairie du Chien."

Alexis faced squarely his doctor, his master and his commanding officer.

"You yourself fled your father's farm so you could make it in the world. I tried that too. Though I failed, and now here I am back with you, my doctor, my savior. *Mon dieu.* Give me that much credit, please."

He held forth his right hand and rubbed the tips of its thumb and forefinger together.

"And you know, I'm running low on money again. Just like you and your time."

PART 3

The Immortal Part Cracked

⁌{FORTY-TWO}⁋

DURING THE SUMMER OF 1833, Beaumont had only the light duty of examining army recruits at the Plattsburgh garrison. This granted him sufficient time for daily experiments on Alexis. It was time he urgently needed. He was determined to publish the book by the winter, with or without the results from the Swedish chemist. He had decided the public cared little about the chemical responsible for digestion. What they did desire was a thorough knowledge of how much time it took to digest Articles of Diet. He set to work to complete these tables with renewed zeal and ambition.

He recorded the times it took to digest an encyclopedia of Articles of Diet: gelatin; rice; sage; soused pig's feet; fresh eggs; eggs boiled, fried, roasted and raw; salmon, trout, bass and catfish; pork; beef and mutton in states boiled, raw, fried and stewed; chicken soup; olive oil; parsnips; butter; cabbage with and without vinegar. He tested aliment via string into the stomach, in vials kept warm for hours beneath Alexis's axilla, and in the sand bath. He pressed on through the man's drunkenness, anger, a fever and an extreme case of indigestion. The ritual of these experiments became so regular that, around noon each day, the Beaumont children would sing out, *Alexis where are you? Docteur Beaumont requires tu!*

In October, just after the harvest, he gathered Alexis and witnesses at Jonathan Woodward's office overlooking the Plattsburgh square.

"I thought I'd never see the two of you again," Woodward remarked. The ruddy-faced lawyer, lamed by a gouty foot, stayed behind his desk. "How was Paris?"

"We kept to Washington City," Beaumont replied.

They struck a new covenant. This agreement covered two years duration, and Beaumont raised Alexis's annual fee to four hundred dollars, one-quarter of which he paid out in cash notes that very afternoon.

Three days later, Alexis approached Beaumont at his desk. His face was swollen and red. A letter had come from Lower Canada. Samuel's wife, Alice, had read it to Alexis. A child was sick.

Beaumont set down his pen. "Which one?"

"Charles."

"The boy born that spring in Prairie du Chien?"

Alexis shook his head. "That was Edouard." He held forth the opened letter.

Beaumont took it in hand and scanned it.

"It's French, but never the mind. I see the names. I'm sorry." He handed the page back to Alexis.

Alexis folded it and slipped in into the pocket of his trousers.

"Thank you, Doctor. Doctor, there's a boat leaving in the morn for Rouses Point."

Beaumont looked out the window at the bare trees. A coach was passing. Two laborers with pick and shovel had stopped to watch it.

"Yes, of course, I suppose you must go. I had planned for you to join me in New York. The book will be published in a month or two. Now is the time to press hard for subscriptions, especially in the cities and other prominent venues. We'll also journey to Philadelphia. That's a splendid city. Quadrilled streets. Independence Hall. And the overland routes are swift and comfortable, even in winter. We'll perform demonstrations to the leading scientists and citizens. And then to Washington. I have a letter here from Edward Everett that several members of Congress will support a resolution to support further research. Having you there for the congressman to see would help to advance our case. Could you be back within a month?"

"As soon as God permits."

"Permits what?"

"Permits me to return. I have always trusted in God, Doctor. And now he holds the life of my son in his hands."

"God does?" He reached for a clean sheet of paper, dipped his pen and began writing. "Each of us has his duties. I'll grant you your leave, Sergeant."

He finished writing.

"With the winds as they are on the lake, the journey to Rouses Point is a day, at most. And then a short trip up the Lacolle River and a carriage ride. Within another day you can be in Berthier. So one month should be sufficient. If circumstances change, you are to send word. Otherwise, I'll expect you by mid-December. You're under my orders, and you well know the consequences if you fail to return. Here you are, Sergeant."

He handed the order to Alexis.

Alexis took the order, folded it without looking at it and slipped it into a pocket.

"Remember, Alexis. Alexis, look at me. Remember the company. Mr. Crooks and his people. They'll be watching out for you as well."

BY DECEMBER, Beaumont was dejected. Alexis had not returned from Berthier, and his efforts in Washington to secure funds to pay for his years caring for Alexis and to support future experiments had failed.

He had sat confidently in the gallery above the floor of the House of Representatives as he watched the clerk lazily announce the call for a vote on the *Resolution to Support Doctor William Beaumont's Research upon the Stomach of Alexis St. Martin for the Betterment of American Science and Scientific Advancement.* Congressman Everett had assured him the vote would be a mere formality. The scene that late afternoon was a dull monotony of passing papers, the low murmuring of many whispered conversations and idle scribbling, until a congressman sprang up from his seat and called out a question for the Speaker.

"Was not this Alexander St. Martin a soldier when he was wounded, and therefore the army cannot rightly owe him compensation?"

Several congressmen roused. A debate was soon ordered. A congressman from New Hampshire objected to allocating public funds for private gain, and a shrill congressman from South Carolina declared that it seemed folly to re-reward this Dr. Beaumont when that man had been paid a salary for his service in the army. Several representatives took to reading the actual text of the resolution. A vote was called. The resolution failed. Congressman Everett urged Beaumont to rewrite the resolution so that it would be more easily digestible to Congress.

In January, Francis Allen delivered a crate of copies of *Experiments and Observations on the Gastric Juice and the Physiology of Digestion* to the cluttered parlor of Samuel Beaumont's house. Deborah held a copy with two hands and gazed upon it like some precious tablet, and then she set it down on the side table and embraced her husband.

"It is done. I am so very proud of you, my husband, so very proud."

He started to speak, but a tightening in his chest kept him silent.

"D'you remember that afternoon in June on Mackinac Island, in our little house, the cottage at the edge of the village, when I asked you how this would end? Do you? I can see that day all too well, like we were still there in that little room I called our parlor. Sarah with her doll. Me with my copy of *Pamela.* You had been working on your accounts at your table. I've long wanted to tell that I was so selfish to ask you that."

"Debbie, please Debbie, you shouldn't think such things. Put them out of your mind."

For both, the image of that afternoon was as vivid as the floor beneath his feet. For several moments neither spoke.

"One thing I've learned, William, is that we really never forget. The details shift and fade and change like so many shadows. Months pass, years really, when I don't think of my lonesome years married to Nathaniel, and even when I do think of him, I'm not so sure of the details." She laughed. "You know I cannot accurately recall the color of his hair?

"And yet, I know that those years are in me. I suppose that is why I always worried about your dedication to study Alexis and our years in Prairie du Chien and you going away with him. But now I am not worried. Because here it is, your book, and it shall be your new memory, and we are whole and a family. You are not only industrious as an ant but a strong, ordered and resolute man. I'm so proud of you."

She reached over to the table where the copy of the book rested and ran the tip of her index finger over the title, over her husband's name.

"And I'm so sorry for how I behaved all these years, badgering you to resign the army, demanding to know when this all would be done. Can you forgive me?"

"Debbie, my Debbie, stop. Stop," he murmured. "Yours are always the proper concerns of any Christian wife and mother. Those years are over."

THE DAYS THAT FOLLOWED were a succession of simple pleasures. They celebrated with a cake and apple brandy. The children performed a pantomime, and the Greens hosted a reading for the members of the Clinton County Medical Society and Plattsburgh's leading families. Beaumont's name was placed on the roll of public benefactors. He presented signed copies to Jonathan Woodward and the mayor, and the newly established lending library purchased three signed copies.

Within two weeks, Beaumont grew restless. He rose before dawn. He became distracted at play with his children. There were hundreds of books to sell. Expenses to recover. A fortune to be made. He composed letters to accompany the special copies bound in sheepskin-covered board which he sent to the leaders of Washington. By the end of the month, he announced his plan to travel south to Washington City.

Deborah twisted and untwisted her handkerchief around her hands. Her expression hardened.

"But you only just returned," she said. "Young Bud has just started to talk."

He continued packing his valise.

"I must go," he said simply.

HE TRAVELED ALONE on storm-choked mud roads and icy dark waters. In those solitary and cold hours, he revised his petition to the leaders of Congress to fund a memorial to pay him for his *"ten years of selfless dedication to scientific labors and for continued support to pursue this American resource."* He carried a letter signed by leaders of the American Physiological Society proposing to establish William Beaumont and his living experimental machine at their institute in Boston.

By the spring, he went north through New England, from New Haven to New London, then to Groton and Rhode Island. He traveled to Boston and inland to a barracks at Worcester. He traveled on horseback with two pack horses for his belongings. He journeyed through mill towns, their massive factories populated with young women and boys from the country. The gray air smelled of steam and decay, and all about were the sounds of rotting lungs coughing like panicked geese. He exchanged quiet and quick greetings with farmers with land claims from the Crown, the borders marked by stone walls laid true and square with scarcely room to pass a blade between the stones. He passed children walking to school, the girls with their bonnets drawn low over their foreheads and their eyes cast down, the boys averting their gaze from him.

On April 18th, he paused before an inn whose brick wall ran right to the edge of the sunken road. He was within just a few miles of Westerly, the town where his sister Lucretia had settled some eight or nine years ago. He rode on. He daydreamed of his father, saw the man at his ladder-backed chair before the kitchen table, the sinews of his lean forearms tense and bulging, heard him pronounce the book some kind of foolishness, an investment not worth the pages upon which it was printed. The price of how many meals wasted? His father told him that a hundred years from now men will still walk the length and width of our land that still bears our name but there shan't be a man who walks the earth who reads your book.

Beaumont's order was to inspect hospitals, and his added mission was to promote and sell copies of *Experiments and Observations on the Gastric Juice*. He performed his duties with double diligence and zeal. His inspection reports sometimes ran to twenty or more handwritten pages with appendices. He counted the vials of medicines, tested the edge of the surgeon's blades and saws, calibrated the scales with a true set of weights, measured the distances between the cots, the arrangement of bandages, the distance from barracks to latrine. He insisted on seeing the weather log and compared the fort's barometer to the barometer he carried in a square box. And at every hospital, he cataloged the medical books, and he made his case to add to the collection a copy of *Experiments and Observations on the Gastric Juice and the Physiology of Digestion,* at a cost of three dollars.

He traveled with a crate full of the books divided between the two pack horses. At the towns along his route, he solicited subscriptions from the booksellers and apothecaries, presenting them a broadsheet handbill — *These experiments are submitted to the public with a confident hope that they will subserve the cause of science and medicine and ultimately become the means of ameliorating the condition of suffering humanity.* At the forts he arranged with the surgeon to assemble leading citizens, officers and others of influence in the community to gather for a reading and discussion of the book about the man with the hole in his side. He showed the letters from Judge Isaac Platt, Vice President Martin Van Buren and Secretary Cass, as well as newspaper clippings of the book's reviews and promotionals.

Beaumont had accumulated some thirty-eight reviews—*Truly a work of most surpassing interest; will be read with utility and interest by all classes of every community . . . The march of knowledge is onward, its progress unceasing, its extent apparently boundless. Every pain and anguish further it. This work is one of general utility that appeals to and should receive the support of every class of readers.* The *St. Louis Republican* claimed the book essential reading in these times of cholera. He carried forty-seven laudatory letters from physicians, congressmen and scientists, and a proclamation from the Connecticut Medical Society that certified him a member and proclaimed that the science of diet and dietetics had entered a New Dawn.

But the book did not sell. The secretaries of the army and the navy, while effusive in their praise for it, declined to honor his appeal that each purchase one hundred copies to supply the libraries of their forts and ships. The English publisher Mr. Highly sent a curt note from his Fleet Street office: *I have returned Beaumont's Experiments, as I do not feel inclined to make an offer for it.*

Disappointments multiplied. A letter dated five months earlier arrived from Sweden. *My Dear Sir, I am very grateful for the confidence you have had in me in wishing to engage me in making an analysis of the gastric juice, and I regret deeply that for the following reasons, I am not able to answer your expectations.* The reasons were many and their chronicle tedious, and the end of letter was a series of questions, each more exacting than the former, leading up to the desultory conclusion: *You see, then, dear Sir, how much previous knowledge I need for entering upon this analysis of the gastric juice with hope of success. As ever, Professor Jacob Berzelius.*

Anonymous critics drew him into a simmering rage. *Medicus* wrote to the *Washington Evening Star* that *Doctor Beaumont did not heal the wound. Does this display of such science and genius entitle the Doctor to a national remuneration by a special act of Congress? There is a fallacy in the whole business. Digestion is a chymical process and no two things are more different that a chymical process carried on in the presence and, again, in the absence of the atmospheric air. Far more satisfactory experiments have long since been made on the solvent power of that juice by feeding dogs various food.*

Others insisted the findings on the time to digest articles of diet were of little value because Beaumont had failed to record a detailed account of the quantity of food involved in the experiments or the disposition and temperament of his digesting machine. Powerful vegetarians backed by Sylvester Graeme took issue with the claim that meat was easier to digest than vegetables. Though some vitalists conceded Beaumont had confirmed the chemical process of digestion, they regretted that Alexis had not been in the charge of a physician better qualified to prosecute experiments and thereby discover what the chemical was. They repeated Dr. Dunglison's words. The book was a kind of diary of digestion, no more than amateur science that lacked a systematized arrangement of the experiments, and they regretted the rigors of labor inflicted upon the man with the fistula, the excess of zeal to prove what a university-trained physiologist could have done with a few well-planned and carefully executed experiments.

It was the review in the *London Athanaeum* that drove Beaumont to argue out loud with the page upon which it was printed. *Perhaps science has benefited even by Doctor Beaumont's errors and a fraction of his many experiments, but the haste of his frontier zeal to experiment, however innocent and selfless was his intent, seems to have forgotten he was operating upon a living, irritable human stomach.*

"I paid the man!" Beaumont slapped the page with the back of his hand. "Paid him out of my own pocket!"

He was even more vexed by Alexis.

In February, Alexis had sent a brief note explaining that the sick child was well again but that his wife's illness now left them penniless and his simple farm needed attention. He needed more funds. Beaumont reluctantly advanced him money. Alexis never replied. Beaumont grew desperate to have him back and to travel to the universities and cities. He planned a series of paid lectures and demonstrations designed not only to sell the book but to refute the critics. His letters to Theodore Mathews grew increasingly desperate.

> *Dear Theodore,*
>
> *Will you do me a last favor, if you can endure the disagreeable condescension of seeing Alexis, to ascertain his situation, disposition and determinations, if practicable, and communicate them, with your own views and opinions on the subject?*
>
> *I would not have troubled you yet again on the disagreeable subject, had not the necessity of the case required it. Not to regain control of or to leave him behind seems like abandoning an important object, and sacrificing almost all that has been done. I know well his disposition and ugliness and hope rightly to defeat them. In due time, he will have spent all the money I advanced him, become miserably poor and wretched and be willing to recant his villainous obstinacy and ugliness, and then I shall be able to regain possession of him again. But I constantly fear he may lease himself to some of the medical men in Canada and so get his case into the hand of the English Doctors.*

You can readily appreciate my anxiety and the deep interest I feel in the case. I fear I am left in the predicament of 1825. I hope to receive the earliest possible intelligence that may be communicated through the military mails.

Most sincerely,
Wm. Beaumont
Surgeon in the U.S. Army

⁊[FORTY-THREE]⁊

IN MID-MAY, BEAUMONT WAS AT FORT PREBLE in Portland, Maine. He dined with Captain Chamberlain, the fort's commander, and the captain's wife. He entertained them with stories of his adventures along the Western frontier, the Indians in Prairie du Chien, and the months in Washington City. He narrated the events at the White House Christmas party, the dinner at Edward Everett's. He told them of the book. But the captain remained reticent. The man ate briskly, then excused himself to tend to paperwork.

"You'll have to pardon him," his wife explained. "Ever since he came back from fighting the Seminoles with General Jackson some years back, he's gotten even quieter. Strange things happen, and he just watches them. This winter whole bushels of cod just washed up on the beach. Piles of them, thrown up from the ocean. But he didn't say a thing. You'd think it was just another ordinary day in Portland."

THE ASSEMBLY at the officer's mess of Fort Preble was just five men. The fort had few recruits, and its surgeon, a Dr. Creamer, was a diminutive man who paid little attention to his duties. The few patients in the hospital were invalids with chronic ailments that Beaumont concluded would have remitted had Creamer applied aggressive treatment instead of his hesitant prescriptions of homeopathic tinctures and salves.

They had pulled the dining table to the corner of the room and set the chairs in a kind of semicircle before the iron stove. At the center of the arc Beaumont told the group the story of Alexis St. Martin, the living, healthy digesting miracle. There was a lectern, but he had set it aside and remained in his chair. He explained the secrets of the gastric juice, the proper ratios of the portion of aliment to juice, and to better engage the men, asked one, an attorney, what he had eaten that night for dinner.

"Roast beef, boiled potatoes and carrots, Doctor."

Beaumont estimated the time to digest each article of aliment. The lawyer nodded appreciatively. The other men murmured.

"And, may I ask, did you have any spirituous liquors?"

They lawyer nodded. "It is my custom with a meal to take a single glass of Madeira. I've done so since I was a young man. My father did, and he lived to some sixty years, and I shall continue the habit, subject to your advice and counsel, of course."

Beaumont nodded respectfully.

"Wine has its role in health. I prescribe it from time to time myself for an understimulated constitution, but we should not think that it has nutritive principles."

The lawyer's great eyebrows lifted.

"None?" asked Dr. Creamer.

Beaumont turned to face the physician. "Yes, Doctor, that's right. None. Once in contact with the gastric juice, it fails to coagulate in any form. But milk!" Beaumont surveyed his small audience. A man who was near asleep roused. "Milk, gentlemen, is, I think, one of the most nutritive substances, for it readily coagulates upon contact with the juice and is easily taken up by the gastric vessels."

A middle-aged man, who had introduced himself as a dry goods store owner and banker spoke up.

"My wife complains of pains when she takes milk. Why's that?"

This was the kind of questions that Beaumont disdained. "Not having the occasion to examine your wife, to interview her, I am at a loss to say, but I can assure you that the answers to all her questions, to all your questions about digestion, are contained herein."

Beaumont tapped the cover of his book.

The shopkeeper was not satisfied.

"Hers though, Doctor, seem less gastric and more in the lower regions of the bowels."

A young man who had been jotting notes raised his hand.

Beaumont pointed to him. "Yes?"

"Dr. Beaumont, sir, I'm sorry I was late to the gathering. My name's Quentin, sir. I live in town and work as a clerk in the mercantile shop. I was wondering what advice you can give a young man such as myself who seeks to make his fortune in the world and what you've learned in your travels about the prospects of steam power for locomotive transportation across the country."

Beaumont nodded.

"Time and patience are indispensable to all laudable undertakings, for you know, young man, if to do were as easy as telling others what to do, poor men's huts would be palaces. I lived for many, many years on the American frontier. Indeed, as I said, that's where I met Alexis—yes, I know you missed that part of the lecture. In such places, as in the cities, there is much to distract a man, especially a young man such as yourself. To speak frankly in a group such as this, there is the lovesick trash of novel reading, the copper-colored Indian, ardent spirits. In those times, there was a whiskey ration. Under such conditions, I found Dr. Benjamin Franklin's virtue diary a most helpful aid for success.

"I commend that to you. You'll find it in his *Autobiography*. He sets out a simple thirteen-step method to master the virtues and, in so doing, tame the vices as well. I did it when I was a young man, a bit older than you perhaps, and it has served me well. With that as your guide and by dint of your labor you should expect success. For this is America. A country of the future, of beginnings and projects, of vast designs and expectations. It is a country that rewards ambition."

Beaumont leaned in to the young man, the better to engage his unblinking blue eyes.

"Ambition is God-given. Imitation of our fellow man is one way that God brings us to our natural perfection. But without ambition, if we simply imitated our fellows, followed the other and such in an eternal circle, there would be no improvement in man. To prevent this God has planted in man a sense of ambition and the satisfaction arising from the contemplation of excelling his fellows in something deemed valuable among them. These are the mallets that break the cycle of imitation and out of that create the advantages we all derive in civilized life. But that same passion hinders others from granting *genius* its due."

He took up the book and held it before himself with two hands as a cleric displays scripture.

"My book is the definitive study of the powers of digestion. *Definitive.* It records the unvarnished truth and, with that truth, casts light upon the darkness of belief. Slave to no hypothesis and free from the trammels of theory and prejudice, but servant only to my honest and humble trust in the powers of observation and hard work and the true frontier spirit, I observed digestion in all conditions, under all circumstances. The march of knowledge, of progress, is ever onward. I have recorded some fifty principles, examined digestion both in the healthy and the pathological states, in natural and artificial conditions. I have procured the pure gastric juice in sufficient quantities to examine its chemical constituents."

He carried on for five more minutes about the book and his labors and the promise of hard work and dedication to a task.

WITHIN A HALF HOUR, the evening petered out. The shopkeeper asked to purchase a copy of *Experiments and Observations,* but when Beaumont named the price of three dollars, the man pinched his brow. He had only two dollars. The shopkeeper looked expectantly at the other men, but none offered him the loan.

"Could I possibly pay you the two dollars and bring you the full sum tomorrow in the afternoon?"

"I leave for Houlton in the morning. Could you get me the cash by morning?"

The shopkeeper mumbled as he cinched his leather purse true, then slipped it deep into his coat pocket. "I can manage that."

BEAUMONT'S ROOM at the barracks was a small, unadorned cell with space for a table, a chair and a narrow cot. The floor was thick with grit and sand that scraped beneath his boots. When he returned, he found on the table-top a parcel of seven letters tied with a twine. A note from the orderly read, *These followed you up from the barracks at Eastport.*

He set down his candle and raised the parcel by the tip of the twine so that the weight of the letters untied the bow and the letters slid out across the tabletop. He recognized several of the senders: Surgeon General Lovell, the secretary of the Columbia Medical Society, Deborah. Others came from authors he did not recognize. None bore the odd slanted cursive of the parish priest to whom Alexis dictated his letters. He sliced Deborah's letter open with his pen knife.

30 April 1834.

My Dearest William,

We are all well as common. I write from Samuel's desk beside the parlor where Little Bud races about like a puppy who is in and on and out of everything whilst his sisters and cousins positively dote upon him so that he is very spoiled and sometimes naughty. Sarah has become the little lady about the house who practices her piano daily for her Papa, and Lucretia has learned now to sing. They ask of you often.

Such is the hasty passage of time. It shall be two years this autumn that we left Prairie du Chien. The roses Mary and I planted last Spring in the south facing garden have managed to survive the winter, in proud defiance of the storms.

The habit of my days is marked by the passage of the mails. I have read and reread now more times than I can count your story of your journey to New Haven, the workings of the steamship and the grand reception at the Connecticut Medical Society and the professors of the college.

Tomorrow I hope that I shall hear from you, and know if you have seen all the latest mighty puffs about you. I need not say how much I feel gratified by the encomiums bestowed upon your work by the public. I see that one of the editors pronounced you a great scholar. That was particularly pleasing, as on that point Samuel was most uneasy, as he said neither you nor him self were either scholars or university trained. May you see all your wishes accomplished and be ready ere long to settle down quietly with your family, who all love you so much, is the prayer of your wife.

I remain as ever, your loving,

Debbie

He sat stock-still at the desk, tears dripping onto the letter, smearing his wife's signature.

A knock sounded at his door.

"Dr. Beaumont, sir? Doctor, are you there?"

It was the orderly. The young man's voice grew muffled as he turned away from the door. "I saw the doctor enter just several minutes ago. I can't imagine he's that sound asleep."

"Yes, coming," Beaumont called.

He wiped his eyes, refolded the letter and then stepped to the door.

"Doctor, beg your pardon, sir, but there's a caller who's most intent on seeing you, and seeing as you leave bright and early tomorrow, I thought it prudent to make the introduction now."

"God, please let it be him," murmured Beaumont. The idea seemed absurd, but Canada was close. "If it is him, I promise all will be forgiven. He shall be as my brother."

The door was now fully opened. The orderly held a lantern before him.

"Are you well, sir?"

"I'm fine. Tired, as you can expect."

Beaumont gazed past the clerk.

It was the shopkeeper. He held forth the book.

"I'm sorry, Doctor. My wife, she says the cost is too much for our modest budget. You know how a woman can be with a man's purse." The shopkeeper smiled, but Beaumont's countenance was stony. The clerk cleared his throat. "I knew you were to travel early, so here you are. Perhaps you could summarize the best and most practical bits into a penny pamphlet? That would make it more accessible to all classes of the reading public."

He held the book with two hands as if it were a tray, but one empty of offerings.

"I think it wise she simply abstain from milk, don't you?"

Beaumont reached into his pocket and produced the two dollars. He laid it on the clerk's palm and took the book.

"Yes, that seems wise. Good evening to you, sir."

BY JUNE, his situation had begun to disintegrate. He had returned to his wife and children. Deborah embraced him as if he were a mere acquaintance. Sarah sucked her thumb, Lucretia hid, and the baby Israel cried. Surgeon General Lovell sent Beaumont orders to proceed with all haste to the Jefferson Barracks in St. Louis, but Alexis had not returned to Plattsburgh. Beaumont pled his situation to Major Pembroke, the commander of the Plattsburgh garrison.

The man listened gravely as Beaumont petitioned for the company and the army to coordinate one final effort to return this national treasure to America. When Beaumont finished, Pembroke looked to his clerk. The young man was sitting before a cluttered rolltop desk; he looked at Beaumont.

"This the French fella who was in Mackinac back in the twenties, the one you wrote that funny book about?"

Beaumont nodded sharply. "That's where I saved his life."

"Isaiah Pearce was commander there."

Beaumont nodded again.

"We served together." He pushed his inkwell about his desk. And then he stopped and let the thing rest. "Other day we had a slaver fella up from Georgia dressed all fancy with a watch and a chain and some kind of velvet vest or something, wonderin' if we could help him gather up some of his runaway slaves over in Canada. Didn't we, Jimmy? Goddamn Nullifier he was, bet you that."

The clerk nodded.

Beaumont bristled. "Sir, this man is a sergeant in the United States Army."

The major cut him off.

"I know what in Sam Hill he is, Doctor. And I also know where he is too." He gestured to Beaumont with his index finger. "Now what I don't quite know is what you and Doc Lovell have cooked up here, but I tell you this. There's nothing I can do. *Nothing.* Can't send federal troops over the border to fetch your digesting machine. That'd be a right and proper act of war. And this army ain't for hire. You want your Frenchman back, well then, send him another love letter. That's all I can say. Good day, sir."

The major looked to his clerk. "Now who's next, Jimmy?"

BEAUMONT WROTE LOVELL a four-page letter pleading his case to remain at the Plattsburgh garrison examining recruits. *I require more time, desperate as I am to obtain the dastardly Frenchman before I depart. Just the other week I have learned from reliable correspondents that a society of vegetarians are determined to have him in order to refute the conclusion that vegetable aliment is more difficult than animal to digest.* He argued his seniority, appealed to the principles of justice and fairness, reiterated the great value of Alexis to American science and scientific advancement. He cited the case of Surgeon Morgan in New York who held his preferred posting some twelve continuous years.

OPEN WOUND

238

Lovell replied that his jar of favors was running low, and he begged his friend to understand the strain upon the overstretched surgeons corps. *You successfully prosecuted some of your finest experiments in the rough conditions of Prairie du Chien. Why not then in St. Louis, where I am told the accommodations are most commodious?*

Beaumont offered to take the assignment as a temporary posting and thereby keep his family in Plattsburgh. Failing that, he began to negotiate every detail, the terms of the leaving, the transport of his family and their belongings, the payment of his salary. And he posted urgent letters to Theodore Mathews and Ramsay Crooks. *Show him payments if you must—but not one wooden nickel into his dirty palm.*

In the depths of midsummer's thick heat, the replies came.

Mathews wrote that Alexis was now a farmer, but he would come to St. Louis provided he could bring his wife and four children and that he required funds to bring them. *You can pay, Doctor, but I am obligated to warn you that the Drunkard might simply swallow the money.* Crooks offered the company's agents to hold the monies and see to it that not one cent got into Alexis's hands. *It will be the same as shipping baggage,* he wrote. Beaumont set these letters aside.

In late August 1834, William Beaumont paid his publisher $437.20 for three crates of unsold copies of *Experiments and Observations on the Gastric Juice.* Four weeks later, William and Deborah Beaumont, and their children Sarah, Lucretia and Israel, departed for St. Louis.

⟨FORTY-FOUR⟩

HE PRACTICED MEDICINE.

Disease and all manner of injury found easy residence among St. Louis's crowded houses and slave quarters, spilling out from the over-stocked Centre Market jail, swirling up and oozing from the open gutters along narrow streets and stagnant levees, carried by swarms of flies. A rank miasma lingered in the pale glow of the smoke-filled taverns. The Battle Row shipyards were choked by steamships' insatiable fires.

Years passed. The St. Louis census takers marveled at their tallies. Slave Negroes, hard-edged Easterners, Creoles, Indians, Italian por-traitists, free Negroes, German farmers, quadroons, plantation owners, European aristocrats, Jesuits, merchants from Mexico, journalists, minis-ters, Irish laborers. The businessmen and politicians who gathered in the elegant lobby of Planter's Hotel called the city the proper place for the new capital of the United States, for was it not natural that as America moved ever westward, its capital should follow?

Beaumont amassed great wealth. Ten thousand dollars in a year. More in the season of the cholera scares. He doubled his fees, and still the sick and worried came and paid well to consult with the famous Dr. William Beaumont, who had written the book about the man with the hole in his stomach, who corresponded with senators and diplomats and had met President Van Buren. Some days he estimated he turned away more prac-tice than half the doctors in the city received in a month. He commis-sioned Hector Berny to purchase more lots in Green Bay. He speculated in land in Prairie du Chien. He traded bonds, bought mortgages, rented lots.

His military duties grew increasingly insignificant. Upon the death of Surgeon General Lovell, he fell into a dispute with Lovell's successor, Dr. Lawson, who ordered him to inspect hospitals in Florida. Claims and counterclaims fast escalated. Beaumont petitioned that Lawson must rec-ognize not only his many years on the comfortless outposts of the coun-try's frontier and his service in the War of 1812, but his considerable per-sonal sacrifice for the study of Alexis St. Martin. His commander did not waver. The Seminoles were uprising once more.

One evening, Beaumont dashed off a four-page letter to Lawson wherein he detailed long, honest and faithful service, at extreme outposts, the fatigues of the predatory Indian wars, and insisted that if the principles of Justice and Fairness did not persuade, then he might see fit to resign the corps. Two months later, Lawson replied with a short note accepting Beaumont's resignation.

TEN YEARS AFTER ARRIVING in St. Louis, the Beaumonts settled at Gambler Place, a mile outside the city, with forty acres for riding and walking, a fruit orchard, a vegetable garden and a geometric rose garden. Their sideboard soon filled with Jaccard cups and Billon cutlery; the mantle displayed an eight-day mahogany shelf clock inlaid and ornamented in the Empire style. Deborah collected silver spoons. The kitchen larder had shelves stacked with mason jars of preserved peaches and pears, crocks of tomatoes. Salted hams hung from the rafters. Beaumont washed at a mahogany shaving stand in a room papered in blue French wallpaper. The bed was canopied with flowing silk. The family dined at a high-polished table with shield-backed chairs. There was room for sixteen. A grand piano occupied the space under the oriel window in the parlor which was kept warm by a coal-burning Berlin grate. In addition to Miss Lynde, governess and tutor for Lucretia and Israel, they employed Mr. Reichel, a diminutive German who taught Sarah piano, and Miss Ellie, who managed the house.

The Beaumonts entertained. They attended receptions. Twice, they met Senator Daniel Webster, and they hosted Senator Hart Benton and Mayor Andrews for intimate dinners. Deborah, Sarah and Mr. Reichel held musical gatherings, staged readings of poems and plays. The women of St. Louis gathered in their spacious parlor to sew clothes for the poor.

In time, Captain Ethan Allen Hitchcock came to stay with them. He brought with him his library of some two thousand volumes. The captain's health was failing from a chronic dysentery he had acquired in Prairie du Chien. The two friends soon fell into the habit of a slow noon-time walk through the Beaumont property. Beaumont's bluetick hound dog trotted ahead, its nose always at work. They talked of their years in Prairie du Chien, the journey on the Fox and Wisconsin rivers, the men they had met. The war.

"The march of time is a funny thing, is it not, William? No one talks of the Second War of Independence. It's just the War of 1812, as though it was over in just one year. In time, I expect it shall be forgotten. The Little Magician Van Buren is washed up, Colonel Taylor is president, and here I am a fusty, musty, grumpy old man without a wife. You read about that Negro Dred Scott? The one in court who now sues for his freedom?"

Beaumont nodded.

"Was he not in Prairie du Chien?"

"He was. He was in the keep of a physician. A Dr. Emerson. I can't recall his first name."

"What's queer is how the papers say he could have left his master then. He had every right in the free territories. Why then does he now sue for his freedom?"

"The times change. I've read that York, Canada, is now called Toronto. We lost some three hundred men in the battle for that town, operated for three straight days, took the ruined fort and the town, only to evacuate before the week was out. Sailed away in ships full of wounded men and tossed the dead overboard. Now it's Toronto. Some old Indian word. I'd say that entirely erases the memory of our aborted invasion. People ask me of the West. I reckon they do you as well. They're fascinated with stories of the Wild West. They love the stories of the Sioux. God knows, they've forgotten most of the tribes, if they even knew them."

Hitchcock began to chuckle until he coughed. It took him several moments to compose himself. "You remember Colonel Taylor toasted me as a future president? Me! Affairs have turned out well for you, William, your practice, your family, this house and its magnificent grounds. Your fame has served you well."

Beaumont considered the point. They were on a hillside. Hitchcock was winded from the gentle climb.

"It has, I'll not contest that, Ethan. It has made me a handsome income, and I'm proud of that. My practice thrives, and though most who call on me know of the book and my reputation, they know little of what I've truly done. The substance of the science is of no matter to them. Few have read the book. Small wonder. I could persuade neither the army nor the navy to see the wisdom of purchasing more than a single copy for their libraries, and I had to pay the publisher for unsold books. And yet they come. They all want to see the famous Dr. Beaumont, no matter that their hypochondriacal lamentations have not a whit to do with digestion."

Hitchcock broke a long, wet report of wind.

"Pardon me," he begged.

Beaumont paid it no mind. "There are scientists who see its value. Just the other week I received a copy of a Dr. Combe's reprint of my book. The man's a notable British physiologist."

"Congratulations!"

Beaumont frowned. "In the introduction, he refers to me as the *late Dr. William Beaumont*. To be sure, he was full of praise for the book, yet he said it did not advance the science so much as confirm on solid ground what was known. For that he regards the work as essential."

The captain tried to cheer his friend. "So then you have every reason to celebrate."

Beaumont smiled.

"So then I see how there is so much more that the late Dr. Beaumont could have done, could do. And I knew that when I sent the pages to the printer. I was too rushed, too eager to go ahead, to see the thing in print. Eager to have my fortune. One of the critics identified some two hundred errors of type. But no matter. No one actually reads it, save for the physiologists and some physicians. My book is just that, a book, one of many books. Just as the sun is but a star."

"William, please, you're too hard on yourself. You ought to rejoice over what you have done, not ruminate over what you wish were done."

The two men walked slowly, each with his arms folded behind his back. The hound circled round them, eager to play.

"Ethan, here now I'm in the grand climacteric of my life, and I cannot help but think of what shall become of me and what I have done. When I was a young man in Plattsburgh, there was a girl I'd spent months pursuing, thinking about, dreaming about. You know how one is as a young man. Hungry with passion. Mad. I can't recall her name, but I can see her plain as day. And when I'd finally managed to get her into the hay, I no sooner had her than I did despise her. I think that it's the *pursuit* of happiness that is the greater pleasure than the attainment of that happiness. I wonder if we ever do attain it. I wish someone told me that when I was a young man all set upon making my way in the world."

He stopped walking and turned and faced Hitchcock.

"Tell none of this to Debbie, please. Promise me that."

Hitchcock nodded. "Of course."

"At least she is content. We speak, of course, but there are many things we pass over in silence. Things I did. Things I failed to do. You've observed that we keep separate bedrooms." He folded his arms over his chest and kicked at a clod of dirt. "I should've resigned the army when Colonel Taylor ordered me to remain in Prairie du Chien."

The two men watched the restless hound trot ahead.

"Do you ever hear from that Frenchman?" Hitchcock asked

Beaumont shook his head slowly.

"I'm sorry, William."

"There's nothing to be sorry about. The last exchange of correspondence, ten years ago, he insisted on receiving three hundred dollars to bring him and his family to St. Louis."

"But what if he came?"

Beaumont dismissed the question forthwith.

"You don't know him as I do. I'll not deny that it hurts to see that the book might be forgotten, that the book did not make the money I deserved, that Congress did not see fit to pay me for my expenses, that they think I'm dead. Honestly, that man's like a hair in the mouth. Some days, in quiet hours, I wish I had shunned the heaven that led me to the hell of pursuing those experiments on Alexis, and yet some days I do wish I could do more experiments, if only to tell the world I'm alive. All do agree, even those who questioned my methods, my ethics, that I proved digestion is a chemical process. My fortune and my reputation are dear to me. At least I have them." He gazed at the sky. "To hell with that ungrateful Alexis."

{FORTY-FIVE}

ON A SATURDAY AFTERNOON IN APRIL 1849 the attorneys for William Darnes called at Gambler Place. Beaumont received the three lawyers, Beverly Allen, Joseph Crockett and Henry Geyer, in the parlor. Deborah rose to leave, but he signaled to her that she should remain.

"There are no secrets in this family."

The attorneys filed before her to pay their respects. The sunlight streamed in between the golden lace curtains; she sat and took up her needlepoint.

"Now then, gentlemen, please take seats. It's not often that Mrs. Beaumont and I receive not just one but three of St. Louis's leading attorneys. How can I be of service to you?"

Beverly Allen spoke. He was a precise man, diminutive, his eyes magnified by his gold-rimmed spectacles, his thinning black hair brushed back slick and glowing with pomade.

"Dr. Beaumont, as I am sure you well know, we represent William Darnes, who is charged with the murder of Andrew Davis."

Beaumont nodded.

"The case goes to trial in a matter of weeks. Judge Lucas has not fixed a date, but we have been urging him to move with all haste to trial. Mr. Darnes is eager to clear his name."

Beaumont sat with his hands square upon his knees. He said nothing.

"We are here because you are among the witnesses we will call, and out of respect for your position in the St. Louis medical establishment and the city at large, we wanted to avoid the discomfort of a summons."

Beaumont nodded slowly. "I thank you, gentlemen. I would be most happy to discuss how Mr. Davis died of the many head wounds Mr. Darnes inflicted upon him and of my efforts to try to save Mr. Davis's life."

"Thank you, Doctor, we want the truth to be known, the unvarnished truth. That's why we're calling on you and Mr. Davis's other physicians to testify about his injuries."

THE DARNES-DAVIS CASE was the talk of all St. Louis. Two months earlier, William Darnes had bludgeoned Andrew Davis's skull until the man lay crumpled in a heap at the center of Market Street. No one contested the

THE IMMORTAL PART CRACKED

245

facts of that afternoon. The politician Darnes met Davis, the editor of the *Missouri Argus,* exchanged a few heated words over Davis's editorials taunting Darnes, and then Darnes raised his cane and commenced beating Davis until three constables pushed through the crowd of cheering onlookers and pulled the man off of the bloodied and beaten editor. The constables forcibly held Mr. Darnes and relieved him of his iron cane.

They carried the collapsed Davis to the lobby of the Planter's Hotel and laid him on a couch. Within minutes, Dr. Benjamin Sykes arrived. The editor was gravely injured with three skull fractures and his intellect wandering. Sykes called for a consultation with Dr. Beaumont. The next day, Beaumont operated, a trephining upon Davis's fractured skull to relieve the pressure. He picked out six bits of skull from the worst of the wounds. Seven days later, Davis died, and William Darnes was arraigned on the charge of murder.

Beaumont and Deborah stood on the porch watching Mr. Allen's coach roll away.

"Does it disturb you, William, that they want you in court to testify?"

Beaumont shook his head. "Not in the slightest. Mr. Darnes is the one charged and the guilty one to wit. Not me. I did my duty and have every expectation that the truth shall triumph, as it always does."

TWO WEEKS LATER, a tipstaff from Judge Lucas's chambers came to fetch Beaumont from his office on Third Street. When he arrived at the courtroom, Mr. Allen was questioning Dr. Sykes about the appropriateness of the operation to trephine Davis's skull fracture. Was the man's consciousness sufficiently depressed to warrant the operation? Might they have waited? Why did they only operate on the fracture above the temple? Two of the jurors had to turn their heads and lean in to the witness stand to better hear Allen, so quiet was his voice. Beaumont waited not more than a quarter of an hour for Allen to finish with Dr. Sykes and call Dr. William Beaumont to take the stand.

"Dr. Beaumont, as the attorneys representing Mr. Davis, we wish to ascertain the facts of his injury, the nature and extent of the wounds and your professional judgment of them. Well known though you are in St. Louis, could you tell the jury about your background? You served in the surgeons corps, did you not?"

Beaumont narrated his service in the War of 1812, his many years on the American frontier, the Indian uprising around Prairie du Chien, his practice in St. Louis. Allen turned to the case of Mr. Davis. Just as he had questioned Dr. Sykes, the attorney asked about the reasons for the surgery and Beaumont's experience with the procedure. After three-quarters of an hour, Allen seemed ready to conclude his questions. He stepped to the desk and set down his notes, then ran his finger over the desk as if to check for dust. The clerk looked to the bailiff, the bailiff to the judge, and the judge seemed ready to address Allen when the lawyer turned slowly back to Beaumont.

"Dr. Beaumont, I have just one question about the book you wrote. *Experiments and Observations on the Gastric Juice*. The subject of the book was a Frenchman?"

"A Canadian, yes, a French Canadian."

"What became of the man? Is he still alive?"

"He most certainly is. The last news I have is that he is alive and well, the very picture of health, a farmer and the father of four children."

"Here in St. Louis?"

"No, Canada. The man is a Canadian."

Allen bowed his little frame. He coughed. "Thank you, Doctor." He turned to Judge Lucas. "The defense has no further questions," he announced and walked slowly to the table where Misters Geyer and Crockett sat, their hands folded neatly before them.

Four days later, the defense attorneys presented their summation to the jury. Deborah and William Beaumont sat among the spectators on benches so crowded that the bailiffs had to bring in chairs and then allow people to stand along the walls before they finally closed the court to further spectators. The bailiffs threw open the windows to clear the room of the ripe, thick smells of the crowd. Young boys and men leaned in through the sills.

Henry Geyer had charge of making the case to the jury.

"Gentlemen of the jury, William Darnes is guilty. He is guilty of attacking Mr. Andrew Davis. Yes, he struck him on the head, struck him repeatedly. This we do not contest. We also do not contest that it was Mr. Davis who first attacked Mr. Darnes. Weekly in the pages of the *Missouri Argus*. Called him a coward. In print for all to read forever and ever. Insulted the man's name. His reputation. Mr. Darnes did what any man so assaulted and injured would do. He could not flee his oppressor. So he fought back.

"But that's not why we're here. We're here because some allege that he murdered Mr. Davis. Killed him. Mr. Davis sustained his wounds on the 16th of February. Mr. Davis died on the 23rd. Seven days after his beating."

Geyer held up his two hands and raised one, two, three, seven fingers. "Seven days." He lowered his hands.

"In that time, he was the victim of slipshod, negligent and ultimately lethal medical care."

The spectators gasped and began to chatter. Judge Lucas whapped his mallet to silence them. Dr. William Beaumont raised his chin higher.

"Mr. Davis died as a consequence of the unskillful treatment of his physicians. This procedure, this trephining, is a kind of carving of a hole in the head by means of a circular saw of sorts. You have heard from five physicians, five, and to a one, I think I deduce that should a physician ever order that I receive a hole in my head by means of the trephine, I should just as soon order an undertaker."

For several minutes, Geyer carried on about the procedure and its risks. He quoted from the physicians who had testified. He cited textbooks of medicine. He read from the writing of the eminent surgeon Sir Astley Cooper. He enumerated the conditions that would warrant the operation and contested each one in the care of Mr. Davis. Then he paused and surveyed the jury.

"I suppose in the end all operations have their risks, their indications, their purposes, and we trust that a competent physician, skilled in the care of his patient, will exercise judgment as to when it is proper to subject his patient to those risks. Well then, who was that physician?

"It was not Dr. Sykes. It was not Dr. McMartin. Each declined to operate. They deferred the task to a third doctor. Dr. William Beaumont. They called on Dr. William Beaumont to perform this most delicate of operations. The famous Dr. William Beaumont, we were told, and those are not my words, but Dr. McMartin's words. They are Dr. Sykes's words as well. In all St. Louis, the good Dr. Beaumont is the most renowned physician. That's what they say."

Geyer stood with his arms akimbo. "Now that is impressive," he announced.

"And why is this man renowned? For the study of trephining? No sirs. For some grand accomplishment with the operation in question, some progress in the field of making holes in men's heads? Again, the answer is a simple no. His fame is for leaving a hole in a man's stomach. That's right— the stomach—so as to use that hole for the purposes of experiments upon that man. And not one experiment, but many, multiple, repeated experiments upon the stomach of the Canadian Alexis St. Martin. For years. Hundreds of experiments upon a hole in the side of a poor fur trapper. Putting food in and taking it out. Right here, sirs. You can read it yourselves."

Geyer swept up a book from the table beside him.

"I have here a copy of the book. *Experiments and Observations on the Gastric Juice and the Physiology of Digestion* by William Beaumont, MD, Surgeon in the U.S. Army."

Deborah gasped. She looked at her husband. He continued to stare, unblinking, at the attorney.

Geyer opened to a page as if at random and read from the text.

"Experiment number forty-six. April nine, at 3 o'clock p.m., he dined on boiled dried codfish, potatoes, parsnips, bread and drawn butter, at 3 o'clock, 30 minutes, examined and took out a portion, about half digested; the potatoes the least so of any part of the dinner. The fish was broken down into small filaments. The bread and parsnips were not to be distinguished."

Geyer pressed his lips together into a simian frown. He shrugged. He closed the book.

"That's just one of many, many, many experiments he performed on this maimed survivor of a shotgun blast. Breakfast, lunch and dinner. Well then, if such a book as this—putting food in, taking it out—confers immortality upon a man, I myself could scrape together a few facts, write them up in a pamphlet and let posthumous time declare my fame.

"More to the point for the case at hand, how is it that a man famous for counting the time to see how long beef—boiled, raw and fricasseed— takes to digest in the bag of the stomach, in a vial of gastric juice, sometimes kept under Alexis's arm, how does such expertise qualify a man to know when, whether and how to drill a hole in a wounded man's head? The wisdom of this book—let's see here, he ends with several inferences—*that the action of the stomach, and its fluids are the same on all kinds of diet*—well, that's interesting, perhaps useful."

Several spectators tittered.

"And we're told there are editions in Europe. That is all very fine. Not only is the good Dr. Beaumont famous right here in our fine city of St. Louis, Missouri, in the United States of America, but so too in far away London, England and Prussia too. But that does not qualify Dr. Beaumont to know when, or whether or how to drill a hole into Mr. Davis's head.

"No doubt, sirs, the doctor is a curious man. Hundreds of experiments demonstrate this. No doubt, he is a veritable explorer who kept the hole open in that man's side to satisfy that scientific curiosity. And I submit to you that it is that very same principle of curiosity, that same insatiable ambition which kept the hole open in the man's stomach, that urged him to bore a hole into Andrew Davis's head to see what was going on there! Mr. Davis was to be one more maimed survivor of this doctor's operations to satisfy his scientific curiosity!"

"Hear, hear!" cried a man in the audience. Judge Lucas slammed his mallet doubly as he insisted upon silence in his court. Geyer waited for the room to settle, then faced the jury.

Deborah leaned to her husband's ear. "William," she whispered. "William, please, let us go." But her husband only stiffened.

"Mr. Davis died at the hands of the curious, eager, ambitious scientist. What has become of the maimed man with the hole in his side? He lives in Canada. Did the experiments end? The table of the time to digest articles of aliment suggest no. He did not study the meat of the elk, the flesh of the orange. He tells you at the end of his book that the contents of the gastric liquor remain a mystery. Some sort of chemical."

A man chuckled, and Geyer glanced at him. "That's right, sir, a mystery." Geyer then surveyed the courtroom.

"Odd, isn't it, that the work just stopped. Like that." Geyer snapped his fingers.

"If the work was so valuable, so very, very valuable, you would think the famous Dr. Beaumont would have carried on with it. Even now, right here at the Medical College, or at some other fine establishment of St. Louis science. Perhaps even Boston. Or Philadelphia. You have been told that the man still lives. Why isn't he here with his doctor?

"It is important that you know the full measure of a man. Where he's been and where he's not been. The things he's done. The things he chose not to do. With that in mind, there is, I think, one story worth telling about Dr. Beaumont, a story about another of his patients. I couldn't bring that patient here. He died in his brave service to his country in the Seminole Wars in the Florida territory, but I have his documents. The documents of one Edmund B. Griswold, lieutenant in the United States Army."

Deborah gripped her husband's arm. "This is obscene, William," she said. "Come. Let's leave. Now." She began to rise from her seat.

"No," he hissed as grabbed at her sleeve and yanked her back into her seat. "Sit down, woman. We must maintain our dignity."

In one hand, Geyer held several pages. He held his spectacles in the other. He began explaining the background of this document signed by President James Monroe. He recounted the methods Beaumont used to diagnose the lieutenant as a malingerer and the result of the diagnosis on the lieutenant's career. The courtroom once again became noisy. Judge Lucas demanded order.

"I'll not belabor these details. I'll let our president's words speak instead."

He put on his spectacles and held the pages before him. The courtroom was still, save the sound of a barking dog that came in from the street.

"*The evidence before the court did not warrant the decision it rendered. The conviction rests on testimony from one Assistant Surgeon William Beaumont whose evidence is more an expression of his professional opinion than a statement of facts. The testimony of Assistant Surgeon Beaumont bears internal marks of excited feelings, impairing their credibility. Assistant Surgeon Beaumont is to be especially singled out for making an experiment upon his patient of more than doubtful propriety in the relations of a medical advisor to his patient. A medicine of violent operation, administered by a physician to a man whom he believes to be in full health, but who is taking his professional advice, is a very improper test of the sin-*"

cerity of the patient's complaints, and the avowal of it as a transaction justifiable in itself discloses a mind warped by ill will, or insensitive to its own relative duties."

Several in the courtroom gasped. Geyer removed his spectacles. He lowered his head and pinched the bridge of his nose and slowly refolded the pages and slipped them into his coat pocket. When he spoke his voice was soft and it was gentle.

"Mr. William Darnes is guilty. He is guilty of defending his reputation from the malicious attacks upon his name in each and every issue of Andrew Davis's venomous *Missouri Argus*. He is as guilty as the rest of us for cherishing the immortal part, his name and his reputation, as more priceless than any earthly treasure. But he is not guilty of the death of Mr. Davis. That event, some seven days after the clash on Market Street, is on the hands of the men who claimed to be his caring physicians. Defense rests."

The courtroom erupted. Judge Lucas slammed his mallet again and yet again. He demanded order, but order was not forthcoming. The bailiff and the clerks looked like spectators to a drunken brawl. Deborah wept. Her husband sat stock-still with his arms folded across his chest, staring forward.

The jury deliberated just four hours. William Darnes was not guilty of the charge of the murder in either the first or second degrees of Andrew Davis. Judge Lucas fined the politician five hundred dollars and six months probation for manslaughter in the third degree. That evening the man and his supporters traveled in triumph to the Missouri statehouse.

{FORTY-SIX}

WITHIN A MONTH, A PAMPHLET reprinting Henry Geyer's summation was published and circulating as far as Boston and Philadelphia.

Beaumont fumed and raged. His children fled from their father's glare. Neither Deborah nor Captain Hitchcock could console him. They hid the issues of the *Missouri Republican* wherein readers debated Dr. Beaumont's ethics.

He took to his study, where he paced back and forth like a caged animal. His dog lay flat on the carpet, his chin upon his forelegs, his brown eyes following his master to and fro. The image of Henry Geyer was burned into his mind so that when he closed his eyes and tried to sleep, the man's round face, the sway of his back, the puff of his great chest, the ringing voice orating before all St. Louis, were all as vivid as they'd been that afternoon in court. Talking to himself, he quarreled with the image of Geyer.

"Using my name like some pawn in a game of beggar's chess! Humiliating me before all of St. Louis! If dueling were not the sport of the lesser classes, I'd have that coward, that poltroon, at fifty paces with pistols."

In time, he decided that the clever lawyer was not the problem. The problem was Alexis. He needed the man.

"You ungrateful man. I wish, wish, wish, yes sometimes I do wish I had never met you. And then I wish you were here. I need you. I loathe you. I pity you. I want you back. My patient, my subject, my servant, my covenant servant. My sergeant. You're a deserter too, are you not? Aye, you're a clever Indian. A runaway.

"Fortune's wheel spun and spun again. If you had not stepped backward, if the gun had been slightly askew, why then we'd never have met. And if I had not come running, not defied the likes of Ramsay Crooks, you'd be a worm-eaten corpse."

He held his head in his hands. It ached such that it might burst.

"Alexis, when I get you again into my keeping, I will control you as I please, retrieve a quarter of a century of my ignorance, imbecility and professional remissness. When they see you with me, they will see us whole and as we were. Doctor and his patient. If posthumous time should remember my name, historic truths will declare my fame. Fault me for my ambition? Then blame the eagle for flying, the lion for hunting, the salmon for swimming upriver."

For several minutes, he stood before his desk, then leaned above it, the better to discern his reflection on the surface of its high-polished veneer. But he was merely a spectral blur. His knees ached. His wrists were sore. His bowels sluggish. His manhood feeble. Life was ebbing from him like water from a leaking rain barrel. He dropped heavily into his chair.

"I'm a toothless lion. I'm wasting my time, but I don't have any more time left. And how shall I be remembered? For the curio shop chronicle of experiments upon the man with the hole in his side? For what I did to the Frenchman? Or will I simply be forgotten?"

He laughed. He wagged his head to and fro like some great beast shaking water from its ears. He reached into the desk drawer and pulled put a leather-bound book. It was the virtue diary he had kept in his first years on Mackinac Island. He opened its tattered cover to one of its finely ruled pages marked with his careful X's recording his transgressions upon that week's virtue. *Temperance, Silence, Order, Resolution, Frugality* and *Industry*. And so on unto the thirteenth virtue. *Humility*.

"To imitate Socrates so as to be *Humble*," he pronounced. "To drown mine ambition in hemlock. Is that what Mr. Franklin meant? To live one's life for death. But Mr. Franklin had fame. Has it still. He is. I am to be forgotten."

He put back the diary. He took up his pen and dipped it in its silver inkwell.

Dear Alexis,

Without reference to my past efforts and disappointments, without reference to expectation of ever obtaining your services again for the purpose of experiments, upon the proposals and conditions heretofore made and suggested, I now proffer to you in faith and sincerity, new, and I hope satisfactory, terms and conditions to ensure your prompt and faithful compliance with my most fervent desire to have you again with me. With me not only for my own individual gratification, and the benefits of medical science, but also for your own and your family's present good and future welfare.

I propose the following — $500 to come to me without your family, for one year — $300 of this for your salary, and $200 for the support and contentment of your family to remain in Canada in the meantime — with the privilege of bringing them on here another year. I submit this, my final offer, out of the principles of Justice and Fairness.

I can say no more, Alexis. This is my final letter — you know what I have done for you over many years—what I have been trying, and am still anxious and wishing to do with and for you. You know what efforts, anxieties, anticipations and disappointments I have suffered from your nonfulfillment of my expectations. Don't disappoint me more, nor forfeit the bounties and blessing reserved for you.

Sincerely,
William Beaumont, MD

For two weeks, he kept this letter secure in his iron strongbox as he debated how best to deliver it to Alexis. He was done with the company. The mails were impersonal. He needed someone to persuade Alexis. One Saturday afternoon, as he was watching his son Israel and his friends swimming at Chouteau's Pond, he made his plan. Since the last summer, Israel had become a man with black fur at his groin and long thighs like butter churns, but the family's good fortune had softened him. The lad was carefree, with neither ambition nor industriousness, idle unto laziness. It was time for his only son to truly inherit the Beaumont name.

The following day, after church, he called the young man to his study. Israel gripped the very edge of the seat.

"Bud, it's time now for you to begin to set out in the world. I did the same when I was your age, a little older in fact, but I was needed on the farm. More than any fortune I leave you, and I stand to leave you and your sisters a comfortable sum, I leave you my name, our name, the Beaumont name."

The boy nodded.

"It's a responsibility I bear and that, in time, you too shall bear as well. This is a matter between fathers and sons. You know that book I wrote?"

"Yes, of course, Papa."

"I need to finish it."

The boy looked confused.

"Finish it. The man I studied. Alexis St. Martin."

"The Frenchman. Mama says he was ungrateful despite all that you did for him."

Beaumont regarded his son. "She did? When?"

"She told me just after we moved to St. Louis. Sarah had inquired about him, when he was coming to stay with us as he did in Plattsburgh. Mother said that we should not speak of the man, for it upset you how he treated you despite all that you did for him. What did he do?"

Beaumont nodded his head slowly. "Your mother's a good woman, Israel. A very good woman. A better man than I."

The young man laughed. "What do you mean, a man? Father, have I done something? Is mother cross with me?"

"No, no. Nothing's amiss. Your mother's a good woman. A very good woman. She's suffered much, but now, now all is well. This isn't a matter to concern her.

"I have something to tell you about that man. Alexis was just a man, like any man, an amalgamation of the good and the bad, the wise and the foolish. I was young, and I was perhaps overly hungry with ambition. I certainly could have managed affairs with more, more . . . care."

He told his son the story of Alexis St. Martin. When he finished, Israel scratched at the fuzz of black stubble on his chin, his jaw moved, he made to speak but then he stopped.

"These kinds of affairs are complicated," his father said. "Israel, I need to get the man back here, to complete the experiments and make my name. Our name."

"Father your name is famous. You're the most famous doctor in St. Louis."

"I'm a mere celebrity."

The young man looked confused. "What's the difference?" he asked.

"Never the mind. Perhaps there is none. I need Alexis back with me so all the world can see how I was, and am, and ever shall be his *physician* and that we continue in our mutual scientific labors. The book is the book. Time will make its truths as frail as dried husks. It is the man who made the book they will ask of, and when they find their answers, I fear and tremble over what they will say. Vicious lies. Exaggerations. Rumors made truth. History is cruel."

"Father?"

"Pray, let me finish. You're my only son. My father left me only debts. I shall leave you wealth. And I shall also leave you my name. You will carry my name to your grave. And so shall your children. Our family's name." Beaumont raised his right hand and gestured to his son with the length of his index finger. "Reputation, reputation, reputation, Bud. It is the immortal part of ourselves. Crack it, and it's like china, never well mended. Lose it, and what remains is positively bestial."

Beaumont fell silent. He gazed at the window. "The wisdom of the world teaches us that it's better for reputation to fail in a conventional fashion than to succeed unconventionally. I didn't know that. I wish I did." He swallowed hard and then he looked back at his son. "Now you do.

"I've an errand for you, and it's only for you. *We have to get Alexis back,* and once we have him here with us, that is the end of the book. I must retrieve my past ignorance, my imbecility and professional remissness of a quarter of a century. You mustn't tell anyone of this. Not your mother. Not Captain Hitchcock. No one. Can you promise me that?"

Israel nodded firmly. "Yes father, I promise."

"That's good. Now listen to me, I have a plan to bring him back. When he returns, all St. Louis will know, they'll see how the man with the hole in his side is still loyal, still my patient. You will go to Canada by way of Plattsburgh. There is an attorney there, a Mr. Woodward. I've worked with him several times, and just this week he replied to my latest inquiry that he awaits my command. He will draw up articles of agreement. I'll supply you too with a letter and a promissory note. Alexis responds to money, and I confess I've been cheap with my funds. That's been my mistake. That and foolish pride."

He leaned closer to his son.

"It's important that you see the value of an investment. To make money you have to spend money. That's a valuable lesson and one that I wish my father had taught me when I was your age. You're the only one I trust in this matter. He'll insist on his family coming, and I'll see that this is granted under favorable conditions. Once he's here, no one will doubt the propriety of the work and the value of the results. The unvarnished truth."

Beaumont had been thumping his desktop as he made each point. He relaxed the hand, and he rubbed its calloused palm against its other. He sat back in his chair.

"So then, son, I trust all is clear?"

Israel nodded. "And what shall we tell Mama?"

"That you are to inspect our properties in Green Bay and Plattsburgh, which you will do, of course, as they are along the way and it is time you acquaint yourself with that business. If you fail, and you won't, she will never know."

YOUNG BUD TRAVELED. In those months, his father worked in quiet desperation. The Darnes-Davis Affair had heightened his notoriety. He had more cases than he had hours in his days, and even raising his fees did not slow the demands for his time. He sold a tonic. He named a pill after himself. They entertained and attended dinners and receptions, a party for Anna Dinner in honor of her *Floral Years*. Sarah's recital of Chopin's etudes at the St. Louis Lyceum received a favorable review in the *Weekly Reveille*, and Deborah's garden was among those featured in the spring tours.

Five months later, Israel Beaumont returned. He was no longer a boy but a lean and hard young man, skilled with money and cards, fond of drink and possessed by a certain tempered calm that made older men pause and women blush and lower their eyes. He carried a note for his father.

> *Dear Dr. Beaumont,*
> *I regret that my farm keeps me from travel for I would travel to see you as I do miss you and your family and would welcome the journey and the reunion, but my land keeps me and I am poor and I am sick.*
> *Your loyal servant,*
>
> *Alexis*

Beaumont read the Bible, made his will, received communion in the Unitarian church, and he began to sort his papers.

In March 1853, an ice storm turned the trees into heavy crystal sculpture, the rocks became obscene diamonds, crocuses froze like sherbet balls. Shrubs were bent-over supplicants under the weight of their branches.

A skinny Negro child wrapped in oversized woolens appeared at the door of Gambler Place and handed Dr. Beaumont a note. Captain Robert E. Lee's wife was beside herself with a violent, unremitting dyspepsia. *She's not slept in a week. Come quick. Your expertise is needed.*

They wrapped the shivering boy in a blanket, sat him before the kitchen fire and gave him hot chocolate and a corn biscuit.

"I must go," Beaumont told Deborah. He walked alone into town.

AT DUSK, the chill penetrated to his very marrow as he made his way home from Captain Lee's house. The slick ground moved from beneath him, and the sky fell through the trees, and the last he saw was the darkening oblivion of the unbounded heavens. The edge of an iron boot scrape cracked his skull like a nutshell.

The constable found him some two hours later, a somnambulant wandering along the riverfront, the blood in his hair frozen like old paint. His trousers soiled. His surgeon's kit and billfold long missing. The riverfront denizens must have taken him for a drunkard or a madman. The constable brought him home in the mayor's barouche.

Deborah sat at his bedside. He lay in and out of consciousness, feverish and shivering. On the seventh day he grew quiet. Deborah recalled the surgeon. He concluded that he had done all that could be done. Nature would have its course.

She lay beside him. She whispered stories of their tender months of courtship, of the sociables in Mackinac with the Crooks' punch bowl the size of a baby's bath, the canoe trip along the Fox River where Sarah saw the bear catch a fish. She read him scripture. She stroked his head. She kissed his brow. She told him she loved him.

On the twelfth day William Beaumont's eyes turned inward to gaze upon his still-beating heart, his organs collapsed upon his spine, his chest rose up like a mountain, and then fell, and his tongue slid back onto his throat, and the little breath that remained rattled as it fast dissipated out into the world.

${EPILOGUE}$

ISRAEL BEAUMONT SAT ON THE PORCH OF GAMBLER PLACE and finished the last of his cigar as he watched the heat-shimmering image of a man riding a sway-backed donkey along the road from St. Louis. The man halted at the front gate. The donkey lowered its square nose, and the gate swung open. The man rode right up to the foot of the paint-chipped stairs. He wrapped the frayed rope reins about his left hand, and with his right hand, he shielded his eyes from the sun and managed a small bow.

"Hello, Israel."

Israel closed his eyes, and then he opened them again. He tossed the butt of the cigar into the dusty white gravel.

"Hello, Alexis."

"Did you hear I was coming?"

Israel shook his head slowly.

Alexis looked Israel up and down. "You're even bigger than when you came to fetch me in Canada. What was that, fifteen, twenty years ago?"

"Twenty-four."

"Time passes."

Israel nodded. "It does. Won't you come in? Please."

Israel stepped aside to allow Alexis to ascend the creaking stairs of Gambler Place, then followed him into the great hall. The place smelled like a shed, and the canvas that covered several of the windows let in only a pale light that made the room resemble a crypt. Dust rose like incense.

"Such a grand property you have."

"You'll excuse the condition of things. I'm preparing to sell Gambler Place."

"It's a handsome home. Just as I've imagined."

"Father loved Gambler Place, but it's too big for me to maintain. It's the land that's valuable. I'm selling the lots."

Alexis gazed up at the chandelier.

"You Beaumonts have done well."

"My father was a hardworking man," Israel said matter-of-factly. "I'm sure you know that."

"He was."

The two men stood for several minutes.

"You're a doctor too, like your father?"

Israel shook his head. "No, medicine was not my calling. Though father wished otherwise." He chuckled. "By God, he tried to gain me an appointment into West Point. Me." Israel gazed at the ceiling. "He was a man in a hurry, and I suppose I wasn't. Never the mind, I'm busy. I manage our properties here and in town. The few that remain." He reached out and put his hand on Alexis's shoulder. "Are you well?"

"I am alive. No more drink. It's still there, of course. Do you want to see it?" He gestured to his left side.

Israel shook his head. "No. No, I don't. Let's walk."

Alexis stayed for several hours. Israel toured him about the property he was soon to sell to a group of investors from Boston. They concluded at the house. It was late in the afternoon when they stepped into William Beaumont's study. They lifted off the great cobwebs of cheesecloth coverings that draped the furniture. Alexis recognized copies of several of the textbooks and the doctor's trunk. He reached into one of the cabinets and took out the jar of gallstones taken from the banker's corpse.

"I remember these in Mackinac."

Israel stepped closer and took up the jar. The little stones rattled.

"Father once told me their story, but I've long forgotten."

"They came from a banker. Perhaps these were part of your father's fee? I remember the first time I saw this jar of green stones. I was sitting before his desk in the hospital in Mackinac Island. It was the day your father told me I had a gift and that I owed that gift to the world."

"Alexis, I know my father meant no harm to come to you. He told me he offered to sew the hole closed but that it was a dangerous operation. He was only trying to make the best of a tragic accident."

Alexis was still gazing at the stones.

"I remember that day before his desk. It was when I realized that he had heard my prayer, and now he was coming back to collect his fee."

Israel frowned.

"Fee? Father always said he paid you."

"Oh, he did. He did. And I drank all that money. Before that, I mean. You see, I had a debt to pay, and I knew that someday I'd have to pay it, that someday God would come to collect his half of the deal I struck with him."

"Deal?"

"When I was shot, they left me in a dark storeroom. I prayed that if I lived, I would do anything God commanded of me. Anything. And then your father came and took me from that storeroom and saved me. God did. He took me into his house, and he bound me to him. I tried to bargain with him, and then to escape him, and failing that I wished I was dead. I stopped praying. I drank. But I had to go on living. For my wife. My children. And now here, even after his death, I am back in his house to tell you that I am free of the man who saved my life."

The two men stood for several minutes listening to the futile buzz and tap of a fly against the glowing yellow window. From somewhere in the fields, crows called. Israel returned the jar to its shelf. He surveyed the bookshelves and the collection of boxes and trunks.

"All these things, these notebooks, the letters, he saved every letter, even the drafts. The books. I shall box them all up and send them to the medical society. Let them have them for their museum, for their historical records. I think that best, don't you?"

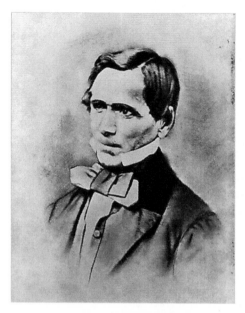

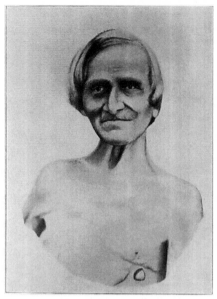

Portrait of Alexis St. Martin, age sixty-seven. Reproduced by permission of Wellcome Library, London, from J. S. Myer, *Life and Letters of Dr. William Beaumont* (St. Louis: C. V. Mosby, 1912), 282.

Portrait of Alexis St. Martin, age eighty-one. Reproduced by permission of Wellcome Library, London, from J. S. Myer, *Life and Letters of Dr. William Beaumont* (St. Louis: C. V. Mosby, 1912), 298.

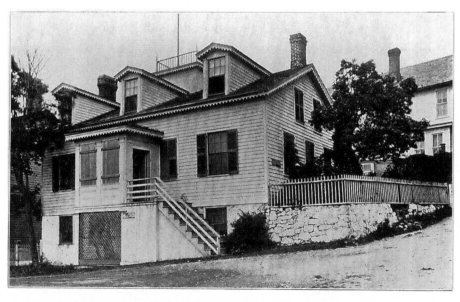

House where Alexis St. Martin was wounded. Reproduced by permission of Wellcome Library, London, from J. S. Myer, *Life and Letters of Dr. William Beaumont* (St. Louis: C. V. Mosby, 1912), 107.

{AUTHOR'S NOTE}

WE READ HISTORY FOR THE FACTS AND FICTION for the truth. *Open Wound* is a novel, not a history, and yet many of the events occurred as the histories record them. In June 1822, Alexis St. Martin, a French-Canadian fur trapper, did in fact suffer an accidental shotgun wound in the American Fur Company store on Mackinac Island, and Dr. William Beaumont nursed him back from near death. Many other characters in this book were also true historical figures, including Ramsay Crooks, Colonel Zachary Taylor, Captain Ethan Allen Hitchcock, Vice President Martin Van Buren, Robley Dunglison, and Captain Robert E. Lee. Beaumont was reprimanded for his "treatment" of Lieutenant Griswold and humiliated at the trial of William Darnes for the murder of Andrew Davis. A decade after Alexis's injury, Beaumont published *Experiments and Observations on the Gastric Juice and the Physiology of Digestion.*

Sources for this book are listed below. Among these, I found Horsman's *Frontier Doctor* quite well researched and written. It is the definitive history of William Beaumont. In some instances, words spoken or written by Beaumont and others, and descriptions of events, are adapted from the text of letters, journals and newspaper reports reprinted by Horsman, as well as from Meyer's *Life and Letters of Dr. William Beaumont,* Miller's transcription of Beaumont's notebook, Schoolcraft's memoirs of his life among the Indian tribes, Beaumont's *Experiments and Observations on the Gastric Juice* and the archives I researched.

Ramsay Crooks's remarks on science and astronomy in part I are adapted from a passage in Philip St. George Cooke's memoir of his service as an officer in the U.S. Army from the 1820s to the 1840s, *Scenes and Adventures in the Army; or, Romance of Military Life.* The list of trinkets traded with the Indians is taken, albeit in an edited form, from Candi Horton's "The American Fur Company and Chicago."

In some instances, I have reordered the sequence of events. Alexis first fled from Beaumont not in the cover of night, via a steamship from Mackinac Island harbor, but when he was traveling with the Beaumont family in northern New York State, near the Canadian border. Regardless of the locale, he ran away. The experiments spooked him, and he was eager to be once again among his own family.

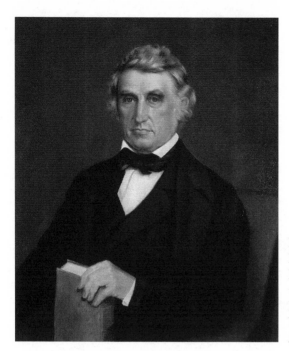

Portrait of William
Beaumont by Chester
Harding. Courtesy of
the Becker Medical
Library, Washington
University School of
Medicine.

In 1826, President John Quincy Adams—not James Monroe in 1823—
reprimanded Assistant Surgeon William Beaumont for his behavior in the
case of Lieutenant Griswold. I changed the date, and thus the presidents,
to move the story along. Chronology aside, the point still stands that the
commander in chief disapproved of Beaumont's medical practice and that
his reprimand devastated Beaumont.

The trial of William Darnes occurred in 1840, not 1849 as I write it,
and the defense attorney Henry Geyer did not invoke the Griswold affair.
Repositioning the event allowed me to wrap up the end of the story, and
invoking Beaumont's treatment of Lieutenant Griswold tied together the
two public judgments on the character of William Beaumont. I am quite
confident that had Mr. Geyer known of the presidential rebuke, he would
have included it in his summation to the jury.

In some cases, I have made up events. No evidence supports that Beaumont met Dred Scott and his owner, Dr. John Emerson, but history does
record that Emerson and Scott traveled as master and slave through the
Prairie du Chien region, at the same time that Beaumont was experimenting on Alexis in Fort Crawford. I have no doubt that Beaumont, some
fifteen years later, then living in St. Louis, would have heard about the Dred
Scott case as it began its passage from the St. Louis courts to the U.S.

Supreme Court. I confess that these coincidences were too good to pass up.

I do not know whether Deborah Beaumont ever read or even knew of Samuel Richardson's eighteenth-century novel *Pamela; or, Virtue Rewarded*. And yet, two events moved me to have her read it: her letter to her absent husband who was still hoping to display Alexis in Paris—*May you see all your wishes accomplished and be ready ere long to settle down quietly with your family, who all love you so much, is the prayer of your wife*—and his entry in his medical notebook that condemned novels as "lovesick trash" and those who read them as seeking "enjoyment beneath the level of a rational being." I wanted to grant her the virtue of caring about the character of Pamela Andrews, a servant girl who struggles to establish a fair and just relationship with her master. If there is to be justice in this world, it shall be made by people like Deborah Beaumont, who see the power that fiction gives to empathy.

THOSE ARE THE FACTS, MORE OR LESS. I want to offer a few remarks on how I made sense of them to create *Open Wound*. William Beaumont lived in an age that seems long past. His medical practice is perhaps the most notable example of this. He drew on a theory of disease popularized by the eighteenth-century Scottish physician John Brown in his text *Elementa Medicinae*. The Brunonian system built upon William Cullen's theory that the central cause of disease was either increased or decreased activity of the nervous system. Brown focused less on the nervous system and instead stressed that disease was the result of either over- or understimulation.

Diagnostics largely determined which of these two conditions caused the patient's symptoms, and what followed was an often brutal therapeutics. A typical entry in Beaumont's medical notebook reads, "*When pneumonia symptoms must prevail, use the lancet early in the attack, epispastics and antimonials*," translated as treatment by bleeding, blistering, and vomiting.

In the context of these kinds of practices, it is easy to measure a far distance between ancient then and modern now, but the more I studied Beaumont and his times, and the more I wrote this story, both William Beaumont and his world became as immediate as present times. Both the facts and the story moved me from nostalgia and curiosity, to empathy.

Among my muses was William Faulkner's line "The past is never dead. It's not even past." William Beaumont came of age when the United States of America had also entered its own young adulthood as a nation. Courtesy of the United States' lucky victory in the War of 1812 and the Napoleonic Wars' exhaustion of the European powers' hunger for territory, we were free from foreign threats. The Louisiana Purchase gave the country ample territory for expansion. Although our Declaration of Independence asserted that all men are created equal and endowed with "unalienable rights," women were disenfranchised, native populations were abused, and blacks were sold as property. William Beaumont was among those Americans who were free to grow up and "go ahead" as they desired, a phrase Americans used not just to describe a direction of travel, but to command action. In the context of this American Experiment, Dr. William Beaumont launched his own experiments.

When I began this project, I conceived of Beaumont as a kind of good man gone bad. I had the notion that he was a selfless doctor, a physician dedicated to each of his patients. And then he met Alexis and succumbed to temptation. A fallen angel. There is a bit of truth in this fable. I truly believe that, for a time, he was committed solely to caring for Alexis, and then he experienced a thunderclap of inspiration and recognized the opportunity and possibilities that Alexis's wound presented him.

The whole of William Beaumont is that since his youth, he was in a great hurry. The passion of ambition drove him to become a better man. On the morning of May 31, 1820, while going ahead via steamboat to Detroit on his way to Mackinac Island, a newspaper reprint of Benjamin Franklin's "project for attaining moral perfection" so inspired him that he copied Franklin's text word for word into his diary. He was yet another American determined to rise up from rags to riches and to consult a self-help book to assist him.

Alexis St. Martin did not tempt William Beaumont so much as serve as the unwitting bride whom Beaumont led to the altar of his ambition. Alexis fulfilled what Beaumont had desired since at least the age of twenty-one, when he left his family's hardscrabble farm in Lebanon, Connecticut, and traveled north to make his fortune as a shopkeeper on the Canadian border. Alexis was Beaumont's means to become a Great American. That Alexis was once his patient completes the tragedy of this American Experiment.

William Beaumont had faith in the rightness of his science, in progress through research and hard work, and in the justice of fair reward in return for hard work. His repeated petitions to the U.S. Congress for what we would today call "federal grant support" to study Alexis were not just to make money. He truly believed he deserved to make money and to be recognized for his hard work and for the value of what was his under the terms of his Articles of Agreement and Covenant.

I feel about Beaumont as I do about myself and others who work to advance our careers in free, democratic and capitalist countries that reward merit over status such as class or social rank. A direct line can be drawn between him and contemporary researchers who list patents among their scientific discoveries, spin off companies and report the multimillion-dollar tally of their grants with the same pride as when they report the results those grants produce. William Beaumont was a most modern American man.

And that is why I began the book at its end, so to speak, with the prologue that reproduces much of the text of Beaumont's 1850 letter begging Alexis to return to him. That letter was my thunderclap of inspiration. It presented me the question that kept me working on this story: what drove Beaumont to write this letter? I knew that in telling the story of his life I would find the answer to this question.

And what of Alexis? He died in 1880. His family, determined that his body would not be dissected or become a museum piece, let his corpse lie for several days until it began to decay, then buried him deep in an unmarked grave in the church yard of St. Thomas de Joliette. In 1962, the Canadian Physiological Society placed a bronze plaque near the site of the grave that commemorated Alexis St. Martin for his miraculous recovery and how, through his affliction, he served all humanity.

Jason Karlawish
Philadelphia, Pennsylvania
2011

SOURCES

"The American Fur Company and Chicago." Transcribed by Candi Horton for the Genealogy Trails History Group. 2006. http://www.genealogy trails.com.

Beaumont Collection. University of Chicago, Chicago, Illinois.

Beaumont Collection. Yale University, New Haven, Connecticut.

Beaumont, William. *Experiments and Observations on the Gastric Juice and the Physiology of Digestion.* Facsimile of the original 1883 edition, together with the biographical essay "William Beaumont: A Pioneer American Physiologist," by Sir William Osler. Mineola, New York: Dover Publications, 1996.

Cooke, Philip St. George. *Scenes and Adventures in the Army; or, Romance of Military Life.* 1856.

Horsman, Reginald. *Frontier Doctor: William Beaumont, America's First Great Medical Scientist.* Columbia and London: University of Missouri Press, 1996.

Hurlbut, Henry H. *Chicago Antiquities: Comprising Original Items and Relations, Letters, Extracts, and Notes Pertaining to Early Chicago, Embellished with Views, Portraits, Autographs, etc.* Chicago, 1881.

Mahan, Bruce E. *Old Fort Crawford and the Frontier.* Iowa City: State Historical Society of Iowa, 1926.

Major, Ralph H. *A History of Medicine, volume 2.* Springfield, Illinois: Charles C. Thomas, 1954.

Meyer, Jesse S. *Life and Letters of Dr. William Beaumont.* St. Louis: C. V. Mosby Company, 1981.

Miller, Genevieve. *William Beaumont's Formative Years: Two Early Notebooks, 1811–1821.* New York, 1946. Reprinted in I. Bernard Cohen, ed., *The Career of William Beaumont and the Reception of His Discovery.* New York: Arno Press, 1980.

Nylander, Jane C. *Our Own Snug Fireside: Images of the New England Home 1760–1860.* New Haven: Yale New Haven Press, 1993.

Pilcher, James Exelyn. *The Surgeon Generals of the Army of the United States of America. A series of biographical sketches of the senior officers of the military medical service from the American Revolution to the Philippine pacification.* Carlisle, Pennsylvania: The Association of Military Surgeons, 1905.

Schoolcraft, Henry Rowe. *Personal Memoirs of a Residence of Thirty Years with the Indian Tribes on the American Frontiers: With Brief Notices of Passing Events, Facts, and Opinions, A.D. 1812 to A.D. 1842.*

van Ravensway, Charles. *Saint Louis. An Informal History of the City and Its People, 1764–1865.* St. Louis: Missouri Historical Society Press, 1991.

{[ACKNOWLEDGMENTS]}

THERE ARE MANY, MANY PEOPLE I MUST THANK.

For assistance with research, Kristin Harkins, Jonathan Rubright, Faye Silag, and Elizabeth Sullo.

For reading, rereading, and sometimes reading yet again, sections and even entire drafts, Hewett Ashbridge, David Casarett, Sam Garner, Geoff Isenman, Bryan James, Richard Kaplan, Ken Katz, Selby Lighthill, Michael McCally, Jon Merz, Clarence Lee Moore, Stephen Reiling, and Pamela Sankar. You all made me tell the story. Scott Kim, your command to "kill my baby" was critical.

For editing, I salute James Beaver, Ellen McCarthy, and Ann Patty. Special thanks to Ellen and all her colleagues at University of Michigan Press—especially, Scott Ham, Heather Newman, and Christina Milton—who championed this book's journey to print.

I salute my agent Ryan Harbage. His patience, integrity, and talent are peerless.

Peter Reese, you are *il miglior fabbro*.

Finally, for John Bruza I give praise and thanks that can be neither qualified nor bounded.

{ABOUT THE AUTHOR}

JASON KARLAWISH is a Professor of Medicine and Medical Ethics at the University of Pennsylvania. *Open Wound: The Tragic Obsession of Dr. William Beaumont* is his first novel. He lives in Philadelphia, Pennsylvania.

jasonkarlawish.com